THE WISDOM OF AMISH FOLK MEDICINE

by
PATRICK QUILLIN, PHD, RD

Artwork by **NOREEN QUILLIN**

Foreword by **A. GORDON REYNOLDS, MD**

INSPIRED BY SARAH WEAVER & FANI'S BOOKS

Copyright © 1993 The Leader Co., Inc.

The Leader Co., Inc.
931 N. Main St.
North Canton, Ohio 44720

ALL RIGHTS RESERVED

No part of this book may be reproduced by any mechanical, photographic, or electronic process, or in the form of a phonographic or other recording, nor may it be stored in a retrieval system, transmitted, or otherwise copied for public or private use without the written permission of the copyright holder.

Printed in the United States of America

AMISH FOLK MEDICINE

PLEASE READ

The information provided in this book is based on the research of the author and is intended for education purposes, not as a substitute for medical treatment. Each reader is encouraged to consult a healthcare professional before using any of the methods described in this book. We do not advocate the use of any particular treatment for any medical condition, especially those conditions which require immediate medical attention. It is not the intent of the author to diagnose or prescribe. The intent is only to offer health information to help you cooperate with your doctor in your mutual problem of building health. In the event that you use this information without your doctor's approval, you are prescribing for yourself, which is your constitutional right, but the publisher and author assume no responsibility. We will be happy to refund the purchase price of this book to anyone who cannot accept these conditions.

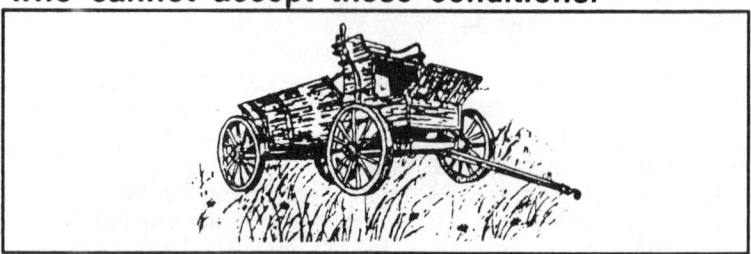

AMISH FOLK MEDICINE

FOREWORD

Nature has provided us with an extraordinary array of non-toxic therapeutic substances. When I began practicing medicine in the early 1950s, medical science was on the threshold of the most rapid advances in its history. My medicine bag expanded from a few antibiotics to include thousands of options for potent medicines. While teaching at the University of California Los Angeles, I found it challenging to keep up with the waves of information that swept through medical science. Over three decades, I delivered more than 3500 babies in my private practice and noticed a dramatic change among the medical community. We gradually veered from watching the patient and using minimal intervention toward watching computer monitors and employing substantial medical intervention. Cesarian rates went from 4% to 35% in many hospitals from 1960 to 1990.

The upshot of all this "progress" was to lose a connection to our roots of folk medicine. I am still awestruck by our technical wizardry. Computer X-rays (CAT scans) provide more information than we used to get from autopsies. Laser surgery brings a new level of accuracy even to the most gifted surgeon. An endless array of disease-specific drugs are available for nearly every symptom. On the other hand, I am equally impressed with the apothecary that Nature provides us in foods, herbs, and other low risk approaches. As I became more convinced of the superior therapies offered by the body's own healing mechanisms, I switched from gynecology to preventive medicine and returned to school. My

AMISH FOLK MEDICINE

eight years as Medical Director of the world's largest health spa, at La Costa in southern California, proved to me in hundreds of cases that whenever available, Nature's cure is the safest and most effective while often being the only option that really works.

We must not abandon all the progress that medical science has made. Yet, we must begin a vigorous campaign to incorporate the natural medicine that allowed us to survive this long-- namely, folk medicine. For most of the world throughout most of history, the only medicine was folk medicine. Remedies will only be passed on for multiple generations if they work.

I am impressed by the research Dr. Quillin has conducted to gather this book. My personal projection about the direction of the healing arts is that we will eventually weave together the best of modern science with the best of ancient natural cures to form a hybrid method of clinically effective and cost-effective means of treating diseases. This book represents a milestone in that pursuit. We can learn a great deal from our Amish brethren. I must stress that a healthy lifestyle; which includes proper exercise, good nutrition, and a positive attitude; will go a long way to prevent illness. Read this book and watch your health improve while your medical bills are reduced.

A. Gordon Reynolds, MD
co-author of THE LA COSTA BOOK OF NUTRITION, San Diego, California, January 1993

AMISH FOLK MEDICINE

(page) TABLE OF CONTENTS:

3	Foreword
9	How to use this book.
30	ACNE
33	AGE SPOTS
34	ALCOHOLISM
35	ALLERGIES
36	APPENDICITIS
37	ASTHMA
38	ATHLETE'S FOOT
39	BAD BREATH
40	BALDNESS
40	BATH
40	BEDSORES
41	BEDWETTING
42	BLEEDING
44	BLOOD BUILDER
43	BLOOD CLOTS
45	BLOOD PURIFIER
46	BLOOD IN URINE
46	BOILS
46	BRUISES
47	BURNS
48	BURSITIS
48	CANCER
50	CATARACTS
51	CIRCULATION
51	COLD
53	COLD SORES
53	COLIC
54	COLON PROBLEMS
57	CORNS
57	COUGH
59	CRAMPS

AMISH FOLK MEDICINE

- 59 DEODORANT
- 60 DIABETES
- 61 DIAPER RASH
- 61 DIARRHEA
- 62 DIGESTION & STOMACH PROBLEMS
- 63 DROPSY
- 63 EARACHE
- 64 ECZEMA
- 64 ENDURANCE, ENERGY
- 64 EYES
- 65 FEMALE PROBLEMS
- 65 FERTILITY
- 66 FEVER
- 66 FISHBONE IN THROAT
- 66 FLU
- 66 FROSTBITE
- 67 GALLBLADDER & GALLSTONES
- 68 GAS (FLATULENCE)
- 68 GOUT
- 68 HAIR & SKIN
- 71 HEADACHE
- 71 HEART & BLOOD PRESSURE
- 73 HEMORRHOIDS & PILES
- 74 HICCUPS
- 74 HIVES
- 74 INGROWN TOENAILS
- 74 INSECT BITES & BEE STINGS
- 76 INSOMNIA
- 76 ITCHING
- 77 KIDNEY & BLADDER
- 78 LEG ULCER
- 78 LIVER
- 78 LOW BLOOD PRESSURE
- 78 LUNG

AMISH FOLK MEDICINE

79	MEASLES
79	MEMORY
80	MENSTRUATION
80	MOOD
81	MOTION SICKNESS
81	MOUTH SORES
82	NERVE & SLEEP DISORDERS
82	NOSEBLEED
82	OBESITY
83	PAIN
85	PARASITES (& WORMS)
85	PLEURISY
85	PNEUMONIA
86	POISON IVY & OAK
86	POISONING
87	POULTICE & BONE KNITTER
89	PREGNANCY
91	PROSTATE
91	RHEUMATIC FEVER
91	RHEUMATISM & ARTHRITIS
94	RINGWORM
94	SEX DESIRE
95	SHINGLES
95	SINUS CONGESTION
96	SPRAINS
97	SPURS
97	STOMACH PROBLEMS
98	STROKE
98	SWEATY FEET
98	THROAT
99	TOBACCO HABIT
99	TONIC, ENERGIZER
100	TONSILLITIS
100	TOOTHACHE & TEETH

AMISH FOLK MEDICINE

- 101 ULCER & COLITIS
- 102 VARICOSE VEINS
- 102 VINEGAR
- 103 WARTS
- 104 APPENDIX A: SOURCES, WHERE TO BUY
- 106 APPENDIX B: HEALTHY LIFESTYLE
- 112 APPENDIX C: REFERENCES

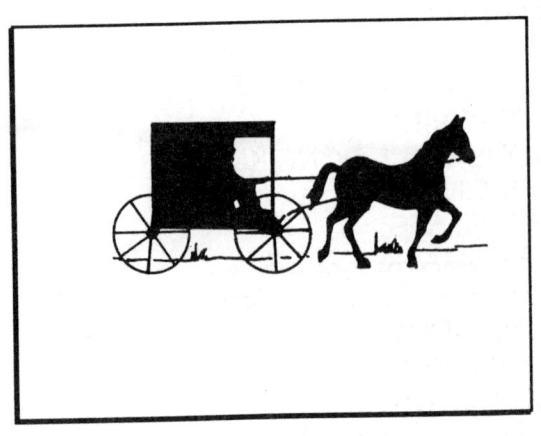

AMISH FOLK MEDICINE
HOW TO USE THIS BOOK
"Nature, to be commanded, must be obeyed."
Francis Bacon 1620 AD

WHY THE AMISH?. "There must be a better way!!" Too many people have said that in my presence. Americans spend over $800 billion annually on health care. And what do we get for this unprecedented investment? We have among the highest rates in the world for heart disease, cancer,

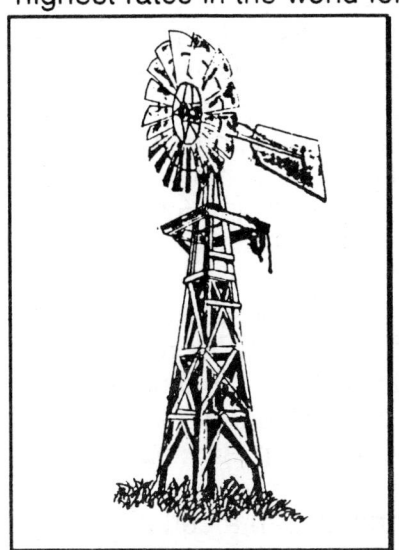

diabetes, osteoporosis, neonatal death, and mental illness, as well as widespread chronically annoying symptoms like depression, constipation, and fatigue. So how do the Amish and other simple people survive without the "benefits" of modern medicine? Why do we tolerate our health care system that the World Health Organization has called "invasive, controlling, and sometimes disabling." Where drugs can cost more than gold, ounce for ounce, with one arthritis medication costing 100 times that of gold. Where the side effects of many drugs can be more harmful than the condition itself. Where it has been proven that a life-threatening $30,000 open-heart bypass surgery does nothing to extend the lifespan of the average heart disease patient. Where a

AMISH FOLK MEDICINE

Harvard professor has compiled impressive statistics to show that the 22 year $30 billion "War on Cancer" has been a dismal failure.[1]

This book project began as a quest to find the wisdom of the "old ones", people who live a simpler lifestyle, closer to Nature. A group of Americans that epitomize the simple life are the Amish people. Although human history is rich with texts on folk medicine, much of it was ignored due to our enthusiasm for modern science. People who valued a simpler way of life, like the Amish, Native Americans, Orientals, and other groups, have preserved these natural remedies out of the need for survival. The Amish movement was born in 1525 A.D. with the Anabaptist of Reformation times. Most of today's Amish are descendents of the followers of Jakob Ammann, a 17th century Menonite leader who advocated strict community conformity. Today, about 70,000 Amish are dispersed in 50 or so communities in the United States and Canada. Through their simple and self-sufficient lifestyle, and shunning modern conveniences as electricity and automobiles, they have become the American repositories of folk medicine.

While I began this project with a certain amount of suspicion about the mysterious Amish who shun society; I concluded my research with a newfound respect for their work ethic, community spirit, family values, superior health, and low stress life. Our current unwieldy health care system could learn much from the Amish. Shunning modern medicine and not willing to lie down and die, they tried an endless array of folk cures to relieve symptoms and oftentimes to save the lives of their

AMISH FOLK MEDICINE

children. The Amish, and other groups, have maintained that health and happiness are attainable only when humans are in harmony with the laws of God and Nature, not in trying to find "loopholes" to these laws, as modern man has done. The Amish try to incorporate ancient Biblical recommendations into their everyday lifestyle: hard work, respect each other's rights, treat the less fortunate kindly, friendliness, moderation, pleasures of family, and sincerity. Hence, we need to credit these "backward" people not only for their efforts at retaining our valuable heritage of natural healing but for their enviable society at a time when the very fabric of modern society is fraying at the edges.

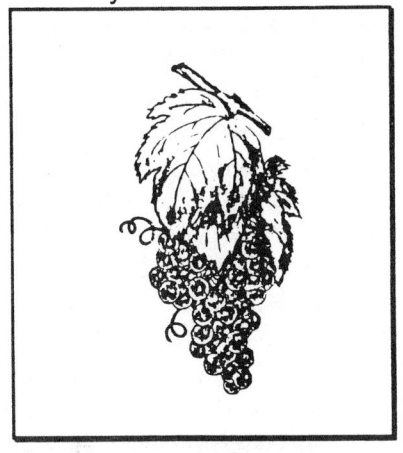

On a personal note, I was having chronic sinus problems for more than 1 year, in spite of trying many nutritional and medical approaches. With great skepticism, I tried one of the cures listed in this book: swab the inside of the nose with Vicks (a poultice of camphor, menthol, a special grade spirits of turpentine, eucalyptus, cedar leaf oil, myristica, thymol). It worked. I could breath again. I had a suspicious skin spot on my face from years of excess exposure to the sun. While the reigning champion in modern medicine, Retin-A salve, did nothing but irritate the spot, a poultice of herbs and zinc oxide (described in this book) completely healed the skin

AMISH FOLK MEDICINE

spots in 2 weeks. I travel extensively and sometimes find myself in a very uncomfortable or noisy hotel room at night with a big presentation to give the next day and no sleep. Sleeping pills left me feeling drugged the next day. Other folk remedies did not work. So I tried one of the Amish remedies: valerian root capsules (3 at bedtime)--and found no problem sleeping and no problem getting up the next morning. For 17 years, my wife tried endless over-the-counter medical preparations to heal herself of two planters warts on her feet. The method used by the Amish, castor oil salve, took the warts off in 2 weeks. My wife also found quick and easy relief for her urinary tract infection by taking cranberry extract pills, as described in this book. I now agree with Halfdan Mahler, MD, Director General of the World Health Organization as he tells us: "The age-old arts of the herbalists must be tapped. Many of the plants familiar to the wise woman...really do have the

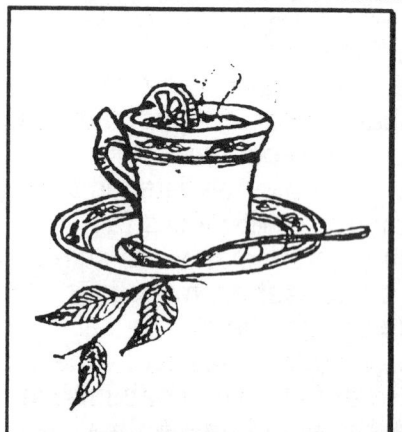

healing powers that tradition attaches to them." My wife and I are believers.

Make no mistake about it, Nature has an answer for most health ills. We did not develop modern medicine until the past 50 years. Which means that for 99.9% of our history, folk medicine has to be credited for allowing us to survive this long. By 60 A.D., the Roman surgeon Dioscorides was the first to

AMISH FOLK MEDICINE

gather notes on the folk medicine cures of the various countries that he visited. Not until the 15th century, was this wealth of knowledge returned by way of Arabs, who had found and used Dioscorides book.[2] Today, the World Health Organization estimates that 80% of the world's people rely entirely on "folk medicine" for healing.[3]

SCIENTIFICALLY VALID HERBAL MEDICINE. Since the days of the Old Testament, humans have been tapping the enormous healing power of herbs. In Genesis 1:12: "And the earth brought forth vegetable, and God saw that it was good." Genesis 1:29: "And God said, 'Behold I have given you every herb bearing seed, that is upon the face of the earth.'"

Multi-national multi-billion dollar drug companies have not ignored the importance of herbs, since one third of all prescription drugs sold in the United States are herbal extracts. Vincristine, a potent anti-cancer drug for childhood leukemia, is made from the periwinkle plant. Digitalis, a powerful drug for an ailing heart, is made from the foxglove plant. Nearly 2,000 years ago, folk medicine guides recommended drinking a brew made from white willow leaves to treat gout. White willow contains naturally occurring aspirin, a favorite drug of todays' pharmacists for analgesic purposes

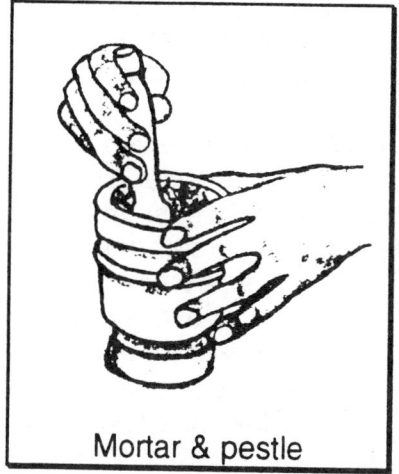
Mortar & pestle

AMISH FOLK MEDICINE

(pain killing). A poultice made from bread mold has been recommended for centuries in the treatment of infections. Bread mold contains penicillin. South American natives use darts dipped in their local herb curare to paralyze their prey. Curare is now a drug regularly used in modern hospitals as a muscle relaxant. Spanish explorers found that tincture of cinchona bark from Brazilian forests treated malaria. Cinchona bark contains quinine, which has been the standard of malaria treatment for centuries. On a related note, as the rain forests of the world are being leveled at a rate of the size of Pennsylvania per year, we are becoming painfully aware of the healing treasures that are lost forever from our clear-cut rain forests.

POTENCY & SAFETY. Garlic is such a potent healing force that if it were not a food, it would take 10 years of scientific research and cost $5 million to fully test this "wonder drug" before the Food and Drug Administration would approve garlic for sale. While there are some toxic plants, most of the folk cures listed in this book are far safer than the alternative prescription drug. For instance, an extract of blueberries (drug name: Pecarin) is the preferred treatment for diarrhea in Swedish hospitals. An extract of cranberries is still the best method of treating female urinary tract

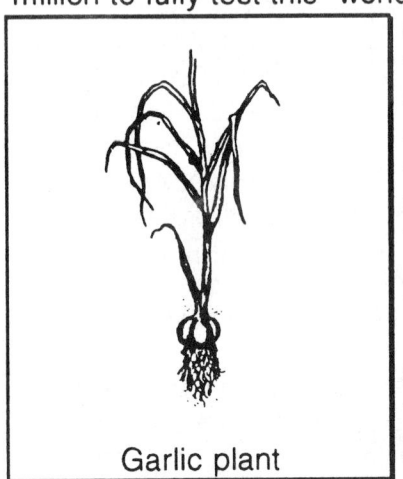
Garlic plant

AMISH FOLK MEDICINE

infections. One of the primary drugs prescribed to lower cholesterol, clofibrate, has been shown in a World Health Organization study to markedly increase the risk for cancer, liver disease, pancreas inflammation, and, ironically, heart disease (which is it supposed to prevent).[4] Meanwhile, the folk medicine treatment, which includes vitamin C, niacin, oat bran, chromium, and various herbs, is far more effective while having no toxicity. One of the ironic situations in American health care is that natural substances cannot be patented, hence companies have no financial motivation to develop natural products for healthcare. Many companies spend millions of research dollars trying to create a synthetic derivative of the already-proven natural compound that will provide comparable health benefits. All this effort is so that the big drug companies can patent the substance and reap much higher profits.

IMPROVING ON MOTHER NATURE?

Folk medicine was heavily based on extracts from foods and herbs, which provides us with the main limiting factor in folk medicine: unreliable concentrations of the active ingredient. No two pieces of wood are alike in grain. No two samples of cow livers are identical in nutrient content. And no two piecies of garlic have equal concentrations of allicin, the active ingredient. Over 2000 years ago, Queen Cleopatra of Egypt used fresh cut aloe vera leaves to sooth burns. Unfortunately, not everyone has access to fresh aloe plants, which encouraged

AMISH FOLK MEDICINE

many people to try concentrating the active ingredient in aloe. However, not until recently have chemists been able to isolate and concentrate the fragile molecule from aloe for more predictable results in health care.

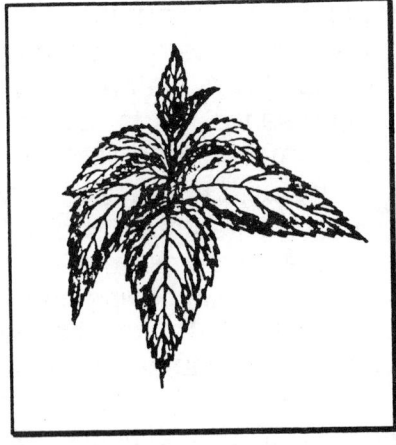

Hence, until recently folk medicine was somewhat of a "hit or miss" approach which worked sometimes and didn't on other occasions, since the herbalist was unsure of the quality and quantity of active ingredients in the plants used. Lacking the sensitive lab equipment that we now have to assay for these active ingredients, folk healers ascribed their unpredictable results to fate or the inborn talent of the healer. We now have the opportunity to extract the best of modern science and folk medicine by using herbal extracts that have been standardized for their potency; which yield far more predictable health results.

That is why some of the recommendations in this book provide for more exacting ways of getting the healing results that you are looking for. Because rather than relying on your ability to harvest fresh ginseng and process it to protect the delicate active ingredients, you can buy it in pill form at any time of the year from reputable mail order companies.

Following each symptom is a list of original Amish folk cures. For some symptoms, there is an

AMISH FOLK MEDICINE

additional "other" section which highlights some equally valuable folk and scientific information that may also help the reader. This book is not intended to be an all encompassing collection of natural healing approaches. It is intended to provide the Amish folk remedies plus a few other non-toxic approaches.

NO VESTED INTERESTS. Most recommendations in this book refer to a generic product, like red clover tops, or vinegar, or ginseng; rather than to a specific company name. A selection of vendors is listed in the back of the book which includes quality mail order firms where everything listed in this book can be purchased. Please be assured that I have no vested interest in selling any of these products. The vendors are listed for your benefit, not mine or theirs.

MANY OTHER POSSIBLE THERAPIES. This book approaches healing from the standpoint of foods, herbs, and other natural home remedies that are used by the Amish and other cultures who shun modern medicine. There is an extensive array of other "alternative health approaches" including: acupuncture, homeopathy, reflexology, various schools of psychological therapy, color therapy, aroma therapy, and more. Each of these fields usually requires someone who is trained in that field to assist you. With the methods listed in this book, you should need no assistance. Check the bibliography in the appendix for some of the textbooks that offer more information on natural therapies.

HEALTHY LIFESTYLE. One expert stated it best,"We are digging our graves with our teeth." Or

AMISH FOLK MEDICINE

the Harvard University Framingham study declared: "Our way of life is linked to our way of death." Heart disease, cancer, arthritis, diabetes, osteoporosis, and decades of nagging symptoms are different manifestations of the same unhealthy lifestyle. Each person merely expresses their own "weakest link in the chain of their body". The Amish live a generally healthy lifestyle: no liquor or tobacco, moderation in fresh unprocessed food intake, and plenty of exercise and fresh air.

In order to make this book a valuable lifetime guide, I have included in the appendix a general description of a healthy lifestyle. Realize that if you are living the typical unhealthy American lifestyle then all the herbs in the world cannot overcome such a destructive way of living. In order for this book to have its ultimate impact on your health, I strongly encourage you to read the appendix on healthy lifestyle and incorporate those recommendations along with whatever else you follow in this book. That is how the Amish benefit most from these folk cures.

As a by-product of their atypical lifestyle, the Amish have far more treatments for bee stings and minor problems of pregnancy than for alcoholism and insomnia. While the Amish are people of a simple lifestyle, they are not simple minded. Modern society has favored the "magic bullet" pill approach to healing; keep living the way you are, just take a pill and all symptoms and disease will magically disappear. More realistically, the Amish have categorized the many forces that make up good health:

AMISH FOLK MEDICINE

1) Solar therapy. Without light there is no life. In Genesis, God said "Let there be light." The food chain of life begins with the sun's action on green plants. Animals eat plants. Humans are omniverous (omni=everything) and hence eat some plants and animals. Everything we consume comes directly or indirectly from the sun. Most creatures and all humans are heavily dependent on both light and color for health. Scientists have discovered a common condition called "seasonal affective disorder" or SAD for its acronym, which leaves people feeling depressed throughout the dark winter months. The cure: full spectrum lights, which can be purchased. The cause: our brains have a meter (pineal gland) that measures the quality and quantity of light going into our eyes. Without adequate light, many people get depressed. Surrounding colors are also important: green is healing, pink is relaxing, red is energizing, and so on.

Humans are designed to eat fresh foods. By processing foods, the Amish tell us that much of the "light energy" is lost from the food. Chemical fertilizers and highly refined junk food do not have this crucial light energy. The Amish people work outside as much as possible to further emphasize the importance of light.

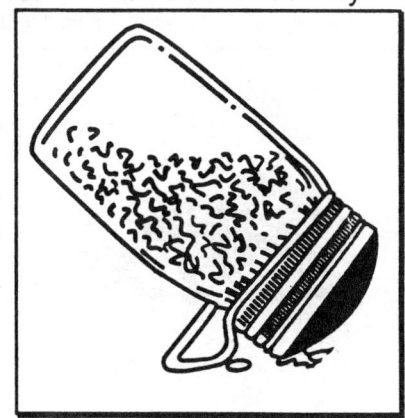

Amish eat as much as possible from their own vegetable gardens. They also constantly tend

19

AMISH FOLK MEDICINE

kitchen gardens of sprouts. To sprout seeds into young plants, get untreated seeds of alfalfa, mung beans, sunflower, lentils, radish, wheat grass, rye, corn, rice, peas, and millet. Soak them overnight in a glass jar. Rinse them 3-5 times daily and let stand inverted with a screen cover to keep the sprouts in and allow the water to drain out. Scientists have found that sprouted seeds improve in biological value of protein, enzyme, and vitamin content by up to 600%.

To obtain more "light energy" food, take organically grown fruits and vegetables or peeled commercial produce and toss them into a high speed blender and drink a glass of this juice daily. Take your favorite herb (mint works well) and steep the crushed leaves in a gallon glass jar in the sun for some herb tea.

Also, the body can become ill looking through the wrong color tinted lenses. Wear sunglasses tinted with blue or green. Use full spectrum light bulbs in your home or get plenty of natural outdoor lighting. Wear a hat in the sun. Do not get too much sun on the skin. Scientists have found that a combination of poor diet (not enough anti-oxidants) coupled with too much sun has led to an epidemic of skin cancer and cataracts in America.

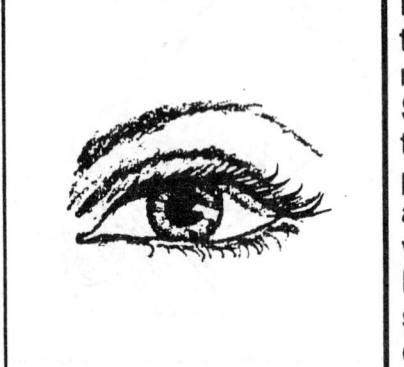

Clay, mud, and spring water all form an important part of Amish

AMISH FOLK MEDICINE

healing traditions. Immersion in mud baths, volcanic mud, hot spring waters, and wet sand by the sea shore can be instrumental in purging the body of toxins. Clay masques are used to purify the facial pores. Clay poultices can relieve sore eye lids. Kao lin (Chinese clay) taken internally helps to purge the intestines of toxins and relieve diarrhea. This same clay is sold as the product Kaopectate. When using clay and mud from the earth, be sure to eliminate the possibility that animal excrement with its accompanying parasitic worms are present. A great health risk for both city and farm dwellers is parasites. The Amish regularly took male fern root and garlic to purge the body of parasites.

Foods that are particularly rich in "light energy" include: sprouts, fish liver oils, liver, eggs, yeast, and fresh green and orange fruits and vegetables. The Amish consume large amounts of fresh fruit in the winter time, in addition to their red clover tea. Winter is the time for many people to fall into a scurvy-like condition due to lack of vitamin C--but not if you follow the guidelines of the Amish and consume many "light energy" foods.

Many of these fresh wild grown herbs are rich sources of minerals: lamb's quarters and okra pods for calcium, watercress for sulphur, dandelion and stinging nettle for iron, kelp (seaweed) for iodine, mullein leaves for magnesium, garlic for sulphur and selenium, grape juice for potassium, oatstraw for silicon, and more.

The Amish slowly chew root of ginseng all day long. There is an abundance of scientific evidence showing the rejuvenating properties of ginseng. Not until modern chemists could isolate the active

AMISH FOLK MEDICINE

ingredient in ginseng, ginsenosides, could they conduct research to determine its amazing therapeutic value. In hundreds of studies well outlined in Dr. Michael Murray's book, THE ENCYCLOPEDIA OF NATURAL MEDICINE, ginseng has proven to be an "adaptogen", allowing the body to better tolerate physical and mental stress, improves blood glucose regulation to help diabetics, elevates sexual function in men and women, inhibits tumor growth, stimulates the immune system, stabilizes blood pressure (raises or lowers, whichever needs to happen), lowers fats in the blood, increases the liver's ability to detoxify, and more.

2) Herbal therapy. The world's greatest pharmacy lies in the humble parts of plants

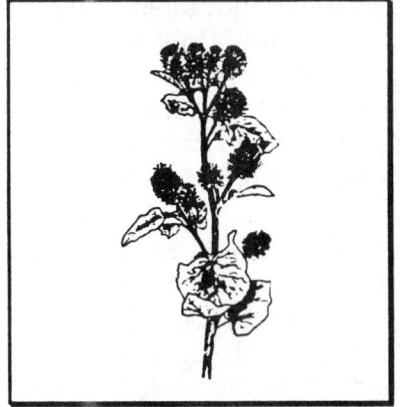

scattered throughout the planet. While there are some dangerous chemicals in some plants (see appendix for poisonous plants), the therapeutic benefits of herbal extracts says that we must pursue this avenue of healing; but with caution and paying heed to the wisdom of the "old ones" who have learned through experience.

3) Physiotherapy. The muscles, bones, and circulatory system are maintained through a set of health laws. When these tissues suffer, so does the rest of the body. Exercise and

AMISH FOLK MEDICINE

body maintenance are crucial. Eating foods that nourish these valuable tissues is also important.

4) Diet therapy. Maintaining proper digestion, elimination, absorption, and periodic fasting is crucial for health.

5) Respiratory therapy. Jesus compared the Holy Spirit to the wind, blowing invisibly yet influencing us quite visibly. In James 4:14, we read: "What is your life? It is even a vapor, that appears for a little time, and then vanishes away." "Pneuma" refers to both breath and spirit. Before modern medicine, people used a mirror under their sinuses to determine death, measuring the absence of breath. Since the yogis of India 5000 years ago, we have known that air is the most crucial of all nutrients. We can survive weeks without food and days without water, but only a few minutes without air. Maintaining the health of the body parts that inhale and filter air is important. While polluted air is defined as having more than 2,000 particles in a section of air half the size of a sugar cube, many cities average 15,000 particles of pollutants in the air on any given day.

The true paradox of life is that we require oxygen in all cells all the time to live. Yet the greatest destructive force in our bodies is oxygen. Oxygen allows us to extract 20 times more energy from food than anaerobic (without oxygen) bacteria. Yet oxygen also causes other molecules to "rust", or oxidize, or change their structure. Just as the iron outside your house is permanently ruined by oxygen, so can your body cells be affected. The secret answer to this paradox is: anti-oxidants. These are vitamins (like C, A, E), minerals (like selenium),

AMISH FOLK MEDICINE

amino acids (like cysteine), and other components (like Coenzyme Q-10) which allow oxygen to be a friend and not a sabboteur within your body. Breath properly and you live, but rust inside and you will suffer and die prematurely from the corrosive effects of oxygen. Breath properly and take optimal amounts of anti-oxidants and you will get all the benefits of oxygen without the toxic side effects. The Amish have practiced this "best of both worlds" therapy since long before modern chemists understood the principle.

Full oxygenation of your body begins with proper deep breathing. Lie on your back on the floor with a book on your stomach. Begin inhaling by pushing the book up as high as possible with your stomach. Then finish filling your lungs by expanding your chest. This is proper breathing technique, which can be conducted while sitting, standing, and walking. It is important to first fill the diaphragm (lower lungs) with air. This allows oxygen to reach the tiny air sacs that bring oxygen from the lungs through the bloodstream to the cells.

Secondly, it is important to breath clean air. Dust, pollen, mold, pollutants, and other air particulate can create hazards to your health. The Amish make sure that homes, basements, and attics are well ventilated. Homes should be cleaned regularly to avoid the buildup of dust and mold. The Amish regularly use vaporizers, inhalers, and aromatic herbs to improve breathing. Remember, the breath of life is crucial.

6) Hydrotherapy. Two thirds of the earth's surface is covered with water. Two thirds of the weight of an adult is water. The ancient Greeks

AMISH FOLK MEDICINE

used to categorize all of life into the four elements of water, air, fire, and earth. Water is truly the river of life in our bodies. The Amish try to build their homes near running water to capture its energy and to reap the benefits of the calming sounds. Taking in and eliminating proper quantity and quality of water is critical for health.

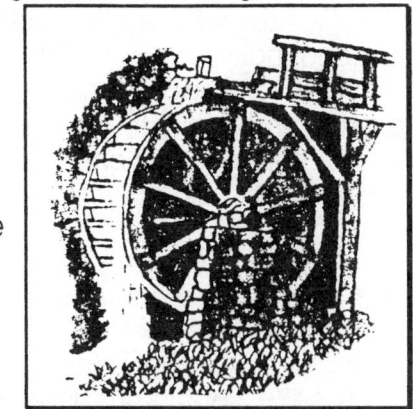

Water is extremely valuable both inside and outside of the body. As a diaphoretic, a hot bath will induce sweating. Lukewarm water can induce vomiting. Warm water can help stimulate bowel movements. Bathing the brow during a fever helps to cool the body. Water is the primary cleansing agent we use to keep our homes and clothes clean. Water is equally crucial for cleansing our insides, via diluting toxins in the body and encouraging their elimination through the kidneys and sweat.

The early healing temples were all centered around water. From hot springs, to Scandinavian cold plunges, to seashore sand baths, to mud baths; humans have reveled in the healing properties of water.

7) Spiritual therapy. The mind is the master organ. Hope, love, peace, and forgiveness are the springboards of good health; while hate, low self-esteem, and other negative emotions can cripple even the otherwise healthiest of

AMISH FOLK MEDICINE

individuals. The Amish have some tried and proven methods for dealing with the emotional illness that can cause physical illness.

-Love. God is love and love is what heals all. This law is first in Amish life.

-Adversity. With a solid community of like-minded individuals, the Amish do not have insurance, because they have a support network of friends and family to care for them during troubled times. Interestingly enough, scientists now find that the greatest risk factor toward heart disease is loneliness.

-Alms. Give away a portion of your wealth without boasting and you will be amply rewarded.

-Anger. A soft answer turns away wrath (Prov.15:1). Don't let the sun go down on your anger (Eph.4:26). Settle quarrels quickly. Resentment will eat a person up like cancer. Forgive others so that you may be forgiven (Matthew 6:12).

-Blessings. Count your blessings. Consider the generosity of the sun, wind, rain, and earth.

-Curses. Overcome evil with good by blessing those who curse you. If your enemy is hungry, feed him and melt his fury with gentleness (Romans 12:20). Cursing and swearing are sure signs of a poor vocabulary.

-Conscience. A clear conscience is the best pillow.

-Contentment. He that is content has enough. The greatest wealth is to live content with little, for there is never want where the mind is satisfied.

-Death. The Amish have simple unpretentious funerals, which manifest their philosophy: "Show me

AMISH FOLK MEDICINE

love while I am living, instead of trying to convince the undertaker."

-Depression. Everyone will at some time face the feelings of depression and defeat. The best prescription for depression is to count your blessings. Amish women recognize the possibility of post-partum (after pregnancy) depression and take extra B-vitamins and red clover top liquid extract to counter this condition.

-Envy. A person who is content with their lifestyle is not easily moved by high pressure advertising about what you need to buy in order to feel fulfilled. It is not so much what you eat that makes you sick, but what is eating you because of what you are looking at and wanting.

-Family. Close-knit families are the rule,

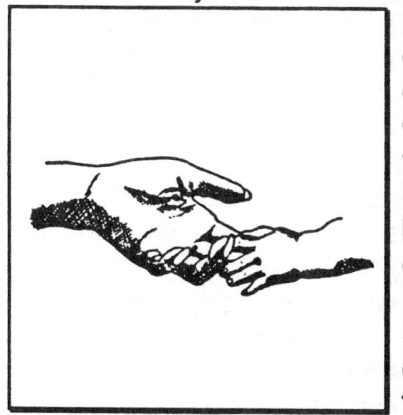

instead of the generation gap and disrespect for older people. Grandparents are not warehoused in institutions but kept at home in their own cottage on the farm (called the "Dawdy Haus"). Due to their community support net, the Amish shun society security, welfare, government handouts, and crop insurances.

-Fear. There is no fear in love, but perfect love cast out fear. (1 John 4:18)

-Happiness. Happiness is a healthy outlook on life. If you cannot change your circumstances,

AMISH FOLK MEDICINE

then you can change yourself to adapt to those circumstances. Happiness is found by avoiding pride, anger, malice, lust, greed, fashion, and vanity.

-Holidays. The Amish cherish their holidays and do only the most basic chores for their animals on these special occasions. Always honor the sabath with rest and praise.

-Humor. Laughing exercises the lungs, heart, and adrenal glands while stimulating the mind to produce "endorphins", which give us both pleasure and good health. Laughter relieves tension and fear.

-Modesty. Outward plainness allows inward beauty to develop, otherwise one acts a part with cosmetics and costumes. "Whose adorning let it not be that outward adorning of plaiting the hair, and of wearing of gold, or of putting on of apparel; but let it be the hidden man of the heart, in that which is not corruptible, even the ornament of a meek and quiet spirit, which is in the sign of God of great price." (1 Peter 3:3)

-Simplicity. Do not become slaves to machines, materialism, and greed. Avoid outside clutter and baubles, so that a person can concentrate more on the true meaning of life, which is to praise God, develop his or her own talents, help others, and to rejoice in being.

-Thanksgiving. It is hard to find a thankful person who is also unhappy. Replace criticism, complaining, and accusations with praise, thanksgiving, and encouragment.

-Touch. An old Amish practice is where members greet other members with a kiss as a sign of family closeness. Many people show illness more as a deficiency for affection. The Amish enjoy

AMISH FOLK MEDICINE

regular massages of the feet, scalp, and back. Massage relieves tension. "If you want to keep your ticker ticking, then don't wind it too tight." Certain Amish dedicate their careers to the ministry of healing touch. Touching is important for human health.

-Work ethic. Parents want their children to be hard workers, producing useful fruits of labor, instead of lazy parasites trying to live by their wits while loafing. Industrious children become industrious adults.

PARTING COMMENTS OF CAUTION.

Your health is important and sometimes fragile. If you have nagging symptoms, see your doctor. Bring this book to your doctor and work together as a team. Your doctor wants you to get well. I want you to have the best of health and not delay in receiving proper treatment when the symptoms warrant further attention. We have a tendency to develop stereotypes, like "everything that is synthetic is bad for you and everything that is natural is good for you." There are many noteworthy exceptions to that oversimplification, including hemlock, the venom of the Black Widow spiders, and botulism extract from food poisoning. Many plants are harmful while some are even lethal. Mushrooms are so difficult to distinguish between the good and the bad, that even experts are extremely cautious about foraging for wild mushrooms. While Nature's pharmacy is generous and underutilized, it also contains some poisonous products that may harm the unwary. May you use good judgment and reap the abundant benefits found in this book.

AMISH FOLK MEDICINE

ACNE

Acne is caused by plugged up skin pores that grow infected with bacteria. Hence, excess oil secretions, dying skin tissue, excess bacteria, crippled immune system, poor hygiene, poor diet, and hormonal imbalances associated with teen years and menstrual cycle can bring on acne. Acne is most common in males age 12 to 19 and women just before onset of their period. But acne is not something you must just accept.

-After washing the face in the evening, make a poultice of white sugar with a small amount of water and dab on the affected skin parts. Sugar has demonstrated anti-bacterial action.

-Take 1 tsp. sulphur and 2 tsp. baking molasses once or twice daily to cleanse the blood. Skin eruptions may increase. Continue with therapy since this is an indication of cleansing the blood.

-Foods and supplements high in iodine can cause acne flareups. Avoid seafood, liver, cheese, and iodized salt for a while.

-Hot steam baths help to reduce the viscosity of blackheads, which can then be scrubbed off or squeezed out. Do not squeeze pimples or whiteheads.

-Herbs that have reputed value in treating acne: (best) burdock, chickweed, chlorophyll, dandelion, red clover, white oak bark, yellow dock, (good) aloe vera, cayenne, echinacea, ginseng, redmond clay sarsaparilla, valerian. Can be taken internally as a tea, or used as an external scrub.

-Take 3 tablets 3 times daily of activated charcoal.

-Consume the herbal combination of equal parts dandelion root, sarsaparilla root, burdock root,

AMISH FOLK MEDICINE

licorice root, echinacea, yellow dock root, kelp, cayenne, and chaparral.

-Take extra vitamin B-complex supplements.

-Ultra-violet radiation, from either the sun or a sunlamp, can kill facial bacteria while also drying up excess oiliness. Try getting a little sun to help acne.

-Some people get acne as a reaction to foods. Chocolate is a primary inducer of acne. Try going without chocolate, tea, coffee, and colas.

-Diet has a major influence on acne. Eat less fat, more vegetables. For centuries, animal lovers have known that the quality of diet will be reflected in the animal's skin and coat. Same for humans.

OTHER:

-Hygiene and cleanliness is crucial. Wash your face in soap and warm water at least once daily. There are plenty of disinfectant lotions promoted as acne treatments. Those with benzoyl peroxide may help.

-Teen years are fraught with stress and intense emotions as children blossom into adults. Teens often develop nervous ticks, such as touching their hands to their face. The hands produce an acid in the sweat which can create skin infections. Keep your hands away from your face. You might notice how some people get acne only where their hands constantly stroke their face.

-Minimize makeup or do some investigative work to determine which type of makeup may contribute to flareups.

-Birth control pills can cause acne. Try another type of birth control pill or different method altogether.

-Oregon grape (Mahonia aquifolium) has been used successfully to treat acne. It has demonstrated properties as an antibiotic, anti-infective, and

AMISH FOLK MEDICINE

immune stimulant.[5] Dosages (all taken 3 times daily): tea from dried root (2-4 grams), tincture (6-12 ml or 1.5-3 tsp.), fluid extract (1-2 ml or 0.25-0.5 tsp.), solid powder of 8-12% alkaloid content (250-500 mg).

-Fats. While 60% of the fats consumed in America are hydrogenated (highly processed), studies have shown that animals fed a diet of 10% hydrogenated fats (the typical American diet) developed a deficiency of the essential fatty acid linoleic acid.[6] Other researchers have found that acne sufferers often have a deficiency of linoleic acid in their skin region.[7] Recommendation: Eat less fat, eat much less animal fat including cheese and ice cream, & eat no hydrogenated fat. Use olive oil for cooking and salad dressing. Consume 3 capsules or 1 T. daily of fish oil.

-Zinc. Among the demands made on the body during teenage maturation is an increased need for zinc for growth and sexual maturity. The typical teen diet is high in junk food that lacks zinc. Dr. Schachner found that a topical solution of zinc with the antibiotic erythromycin was very effective at healing acne.[8] Oral zinc supplements also healed acne.[9] In a particularly impressive experiment, 58% of acne subjects taking oral zinc supplements received marked improvement in their condition while none of the placebo group had any improvement.[10] Recommendations: take 50-100 mg/day of zinc picolinate (a very well absorbed form of zinc).

-Vitamin A works in many different systems in the body, including maintaining the health of the skin. Research has shown that high doses of vitamin A

improve acne.[11] Recommendation: eat 3 ounces of liver at least once each week plus more green and orange fruits and vegetables (rich in beta-carotene form of A), plus take 25,000 iu of beta-carotene and 5,000 iu of vitamin A each day as pill supplements.
-Chromium is an essential mineral that is involved in processing sugar in the bloodstream. Chromium from brewer's yeast was scientifically proven to treat acne in 9 human subjects.[12] Recommendation: take 400 mcg/day of chromium as chromium picolinate (very absorbable) or 2 tsp. of high chromium yeast.
-Vitamin E & selenium. These two essential nutrients work in conjunction to create an important protective enzyme in the body, called glutathione peroxidase. Six weeks of therapy with 400 mcg of selenium and 30 iu of vitamin E helped the majority of the 29 acne patients in this study.[13]

AGE SPOTS

As we age, the processes of living take their toll and accumulate cellular debris, often called age spots. In some people, the liver is so undernourished or overwhelmed with toxins that it cannot excrete these waste products. Or, lack of anti-oxidants to slow the "rusting" process of aging causes buildup of age spots. Life is basically an endless series of "bringing in the groceries" (i.e. eating the right nutrients to feed the cells) and "taking out the trash" (i.e. excreting the waste products that are a natural by-product of living). If your body is not efficiently "taking out the trash" or bringing in the right groceries, then age spots occur.
-Herbs that may help include: dandelion, ginseng, gotu kola, licorice sarsaparilla.

OTHER:
-Bilberry (Vaccinium myrtillus) has been shown to slow many of the processes of aging, act as an antioxidant, stabilizes connection tissue (collagen), strengthens and stabilizes blood vessels, and improves other side effects of aging.
Recommendations: 4-8 ounces daily of fresh berries, or bilberry extract at 25% anthocyanidin taking 80-160 mg, or anthocyanosides at 20-40 mg/day.
-Aging is a normal function of living, while premature aging is an accumulation of decades of neglect or abuse. It is oxidation that encourages early destruction of tissue that leads to cataracts, blocked vessels, inoperable minds, and cancer. Use the overall healthy lifestyle and daily intake of antioxidants as described in the appendix.[14]

ALCOHOLISM
-Abstinence is the best method for prevention of the problem
-Swallow 1 T. pure olive oil before drinking to relieve the cravings.
OTHER:
-There is substantial evidence that amino acids, or the building blocks that make up proteins, can provide relief from the craving for alcohol.
Recommendations: take 5 grams daily of L-glutamine, 2 grams of L-tryptophan, 3-4 grams of gamma-hydroxybutyric acid, 2 grams fish and borage oil emulsion (eicosapentaenoic acid plus gamma-linolenic acid) from BioSyn, 1 gram pantethine, plus avoidance of sugar and caffeine to help stabilize blood sugar levels.[15]

AMISH FOLK MEDICINE

-One of the most productive nutrition scientists of the 20th century was Dr. Roger Williams of the University of Texas. Dr. Williams gathered data into a book showing that alcoholism can be a manifestation of unmet nutrient requirements. With the complexities of the human body and diet, there are no "magic bullet" nutrients but rather a total approach to satisfying the biochemical needs of the body. His book is highly recommended[16] and closely follows the appendix section on "healthy lifestyle."

ALLERGIES
-Chew honeycomb honey to help dry up runny nose and unblock congested sinuses.
-Cleanse the sinuses with warm salt water. Prepare

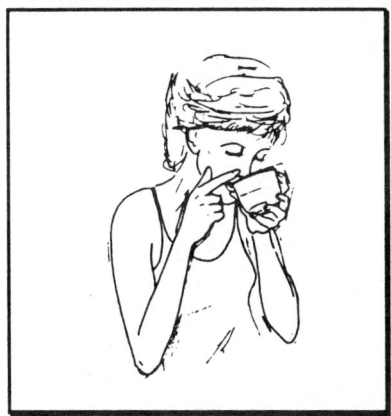

a solution using 1/2 tsp. salt (preferably sea salt) mixed in 8 ounces of filtered warm water. Bend over the sink and slowly inhale through the nose, drawing the salt water solution into the sinuses. Plug your nose with your fingers to allow the solution to soak inside the sinuses. Breath through the mouth and hold water in sinuses for about 20 seconds. Expel the solution along with any mucous and debris. Continue this process until the sinuses have been cleansed. A saving ritual for people who work around dust and sawdust. Helps to reduce time spent with a cold. Also, helpful for bad breath and allergies.

AMISH FOLK MEDICINE

OTHER:
-Tape or tie a small amount of food, dust, or whatever you think may be causing your allergy to your skin and leave it for 24 hours. If a red spot or rash appears, then you are probably allergic to that substance.
-Allergies can be caused by tension, emotion, toxic burden, or undigested protein particles.
-Your body's allergic reactions are an over-response by the immune system. One way to help subdue the symptoms of an allergy is to take vitamin C to suppress the release of histamines.
Recommendations: start by taking 2 grams/day of ascorbic acid, then adding 1 gram extra each day until you are taking 12 gram/day. Use 2 grams or less for children under 5 years. Use a buffered form of C if digestive problems develop. Easiest and cheapest way to increase C intake is by using powdered form as 1 tsp. (contains 4 grams) in a small glass of fruit juice, taken 3 times daily (total=12 grams). Follow the other guidelines for healthy lifestyle in the appendix.
-Allergies can be caused by incomplete digestion of proteins (therefore take 3 digestive enzyme tablets at each meal), or by low thyroid output (therefore take thyroid replacement medication), or by stress (therefore reduce or avoid stressors), or calcium/magnesium deficiencies, etc.[17]

APPENDICITIS

The appendix is a small finger-like projection from the intestines which is an active part of digestion in rabbits and other herbivores but is inactive in humans. This little side spur detour can accumulate

AMISH FOLK MEDICINE

debris which can become inflamed and infected. A burst appendix can be lethal, since the bacteria spills into the abdominal cavity and bloodstream. Seek medical attention promptly if you think the appendix is inflamed.
-One tsp. of flaxseed daily may prevent the problem.
-One tsp. of olive oil daily may prevent the problem.
-Roughage in the diet may prevent the problem.
    OTHER:
-People on low fiber diets are more likely to develop appendicitis.

ASTHMA

Asthma involves a reduction in the flow of air to the lungs. The bronchial tubes leading to the lungs can be constricted or inflamed, giving the person the feeling of suffocating.
-Avoid dusty, smokey, dirty air environments; especially for children.
-Drink tea from Breath Easy tea brand, found in health food stores.
-Formulate a syrup from comfrey root, mullein, garlic, fennel seed, and lobelia in vegetable glycerine and apple cider vinegar.
-Take 4 T. aloe vera gel before meals and at bedtime (4 times daily) for 2 weeks.
-To relieve an asthma attack, steep 4 oz. powdered lobelia in 1 quart rum, let stand for 1 week, then strain. Take 1/2 tsp. this solution during an attack or use 3 drops 3 times daily as a preventive measure.
-Many asthma attacks are incited by food allergies. Eliminate all highly refined foods: sugar, white flour, homogenized whole milk, coffee, black tea, soda pop, chocolate.

AMISH FOLK MEDICINE

-Take 3 capsules 3 times daily of equal parts: marshmallow, mullein, comfrey, lobelia, and chickweed.
-For deep bronchial coughs, chew on peeled ginseng root.
-Ten drops 3 times daily of elderberry tincture helps coughs.
-Mix the following herbal ingredients: 3 parts coughwart, 3 parts sage, 3 parts plantain, 1 part mullein. Add 1 c. boiling water, cool, then strain. Take one tsp. of this fluid every hour.
-Mullein leaf (Aaron's rod) tea may be helpful.
-To relieve the suffocating feeling, press a very cold, wet rag against the forehead.
    OTHER:
-Food allergies are often the cause of asthma.[18]
-Food additives, such as metabisulfite or monosodium glutamate, can cause asthma.[19]
-Vitamin B-6 supplements (50-100 mg/day) have been shown to reduce the incidence and severity of childhood asthma attacks.[20]
-Vitamin C supplements (1-2 grams/day) can reduce asthma attacks by lowering the sensitivity of the asthmatic person.[21]
-Magnesium supplements (400-800 mg/day) have reduced the severity of asthma attacks in human subjects.[22]

ATHLETE'S FOOT (or Foot Fungus.)

This common condition is basically a fungal infection that thrives on warm, moist, dark places; like the places between toes. Among the simple ways of making life tough on this fungus is to change the pH

AMISH FOLK MEDICINE

(acid/base balance) by soaking the feet in a solution of mild acid (like vinegar) or alkaline (like baking soda).
-To a bowl of very warm water, add 1/2 c. of vinegar and soak feet. Repeat daily.
-Apply undesine ointment, available wherever herbs and natural remedies are sold.
-Sprinkle baking soda in bottom of shoes, on feet, and in socks. Repeat daily. Very helpful for sweaty and/or smelly feet.
-Apply the raw juice from jewelweed (touch-me-not).
-Apply a salve of lard, iodine, powdered egg shells, and sulphur.
-Wash feet often in a mild solution of boric acid.
-Rinse feet in tea made from jewelweed, nasturtium, and muskmelon.
    OTHER:
-Daily supplements of garlic (6-8 capsules) and Lactobacillus pills or yogurt will bolster the immune system to ward off this fungal infection.[23]

BAD BREATH

    Bad breath usually stems from either the sinuses or the stomach. If your sinuses are plugged, irritated, or infected; then see the allergy section.
-Chew anise seeds after meal.
-Pare off root bark of sweet calamus, then chew inside "meat".
-Take 5 grams daily of purified charcoal tablets to cleanse the stomach and intestines.
-Stomach problems can be caused by a multitude of lifestyle factors: stress, liquor, overeating, high fat meals, insufficient supply of digestive enzymes, etc.

AMISH FOLK MEDICINE

-Eat less fat and sugar while consuming more green vegetables, like spinach, kale, collards, beet greens, and broccoli.
-Peppermint tea helps a "sour" stomach.
-An herbal concoction composed of peppermint, Gentian root, goldenseal root, atractylodes root, dandelion root, licorice root, anise seed, burdock root, ginger root, and fennel seed is available from Zand Formulas and called Digest Herbal.
   OTHER:
-For indigestion, avoid foods high in fat, spices, and milk curd (such as pizza). Take digestive enzymes (2-4 tablets with each meal), the herb Gentian Lutea (1-2 grams dried rhizome & roots), hydrochloric acid tablets (one 10 grain tablet per meal, then build up to "warm" feeling in stomach, then cut back), and eat more kiwi, papaya, and pineapple (all contain digestive enzymes).[24]

BALDNESS (see "hair & skin care")

BATH (hydrotherapy)
-Take a relaxaing bath with the following herbs added: rose petals, mint leaves, sweet marjoram, lemon balm, verbena, lavender.
-Add 1 c. epsom salts to a hot bath and soak for 15 minutes for healthy detoxification.
-For aching muscles, add 2 T. dry mustard powder to hot bath and soak for 15 minutes.
-To help eliminate perspiration odors, add 1/2 c. bicarbonate of soda to hot bath.

BEDSORES

AMISH FOLK MEDICINE

People who are confined to bed for long periods of time have a tendency to develop sores, pimples, open wounds, and other signs of skin breakdown. Much of these problems are due to poor circulation.
-Mix white sugar with an unbeaten egg white and apply to sore.
-Mix 1 tsp. white sugar with milk of magnesia and hydrogen peroxide to form a poultice. Apply to sores and cover with bandage.
-Soak towels in warm epsom salts and lay on sore. Once the towel cools, apply a poultice plaster of clay pine.
-Make a salve from 1/2 oz. oil of wintergreen, 1 oz. glycerine, 2 oz. of rubbing alcohol, 2 oz. water.
-Omit food high in fat, sugar, and salt from the diet to improve the comfort of the patient.
-Apply Preparation H to sores.
   OTHER:
-Use a special bed that provides either a variable firmness mattress, or a foam mattress topper that encourages better circulation in the skin (such as sheepskin).
-Move or roll over as much as possible. Lying in one position for long periods of time nearly guarantees bedsores.

BEDWETTING

While we sleep, most people have the autonomic nervous and muscular development to keep the bladder muscles tight. Bedwetters often grow out of this symptom as they mature. Yet many methods show that bedwetting after age 3 or 4 is easily treated.

AMISH FOLK MEDICINE

-Bedwetting is often caused by deep sleeping. Set an alarm clock for the bedwetter to get up every 3 hours and urinate.
-Give the person 1-2 tsp. of honey before retiring.
-Avoid intake of fluids after 5 pm.
-Drink a solution of 1 tsp. epsom salts dissolved in 8 oz. water with each noon meal.
-Eat dandelion plant and root. The roots can be cut up and roasted for a coffee substitute.
　OTHER:
-Bedwetting is another symptom of allergies[25]. By finding the offending food, the bedwetting often stops. Mostly likely food suspects: milk and other dairy products, wheat, and beef. Refer to HEALING NUTRIENTS (see bibliography) for the chapter on isolating food allergies.

BLEEDING

　　　The clotting ability of our blood depends on a number of factors that influence "prostaglandin" production. Prostaglandins are extremely potent substances in the body which regulate everything from muscle contractions, to immune activity, to the clotting ability of the blood supply. Of course, excessive bleeding can be fatal and requires medical attention.
-Use tincture of boiled clover blossoms to bath fresh wounds and sores.
-If someone has just stepped on a nail or pitchfork, soak the foot in a bucket of warm water to which a handful of wood ashes has been added. Make sure that you have had a tetanus shot within 2 years.
-Soak fresh wounds that have closed in saffron tea for rapid healing.

AMISH FOLK MEDICINE

-Apply a poultice of grated onion to a fresh wound or cut.
-Wash off bleeding sores with pure vinegar to help the blood coagulate.
-Apply powdered alum to cuts to cause the skin to close.
-Cover the cut with unglazed brown paper bag wet with vinegar.
-Apply powdered cayenne pepper to the wound.
-Clean first with hydrogen peroxide before trying to close the wound.
   OTHER:
-Vitamin K deficiency can cause excess bleeding. Best sources of vitamin K are green and orange vegetables, liver, and stimulating the growth of healthy intestinal bacteria by eating yogurt.[26]
-Poor clotting can be cause by excess consumption of aspirin, fish oil, or the use of anti-coagulant drugs given to heart disease patients

BLOOD CLOTS

In the typical modern lifestyle, the blood has a tendency to become sticky and clump together, which creates numerous problems. Clots (thrombus) can get wedged in veins of the legs (phlebitis) or brain (stroke). Sticky blood is indicative of a very serious problem, not just an inconvenient symptom. See your doctor.

-Take a few drops of juniper oil daily.
   OTHER:
-The stickiness of the blood is highly dependent on a set of body substances called prostaglandins. When we eat more sugar, saturated fat, hydrogenated fat, coupled with low intake of vitamin E; we are creating sticky blood cells that clot when they shouldn't. Eat

AMISH FOLK MEDICINE

sweets in moderation and only with a mixed meal of protein, fat, and complex carbohydrates. Take 3-9 capsules/day of fish oil, or 1-3 T. of liquid fish oil to markedly reduce the stickiness of blood cells.[27] Take 2400 iu/day of mixed natural tocopherols of vitamin E from Grace Company (see appendix).
-While there are numerous studies showing that 1-2 aspirin/day can reduce the stickiness of blood cells and hence the risk for cancer or heart disease; there are an equal number of studies showing that aspirin has many side effects, including intestinal bleeding which make it far from the "safe" drug it is called. I do not encourage the long term use of aspirin as a preventive agent.

BLOOD BUILDER (ANEMIA)

One of the most common malnutritive conditions in the world is iron deficiency anemia. Since iron is needed to make healthy red blood cells to deliver oxygen to all cells in the body, iron deficiency symptoms read more like a patient who is slowly suffocating; including fatigue, lethary, confusion, irritability, gray skin (in extreme stages), and frequent infections.
-Take a drink made from 1 part red beet juice to 2 parts red grape juice. Take 1 T. 3-4 times daily. As a substitute, take beet powder capsules.
    OTHER:
-The building of adequate red blood cells involves a host of nutrients, including daily supplies of iron (10-30 mg), zinc (10-50 mg), copper (1-5 mg), B-12 (100-3000 mcg, may need to be intravenous or sublingual), folate (400-800 mcg), B-6 (5-50 mg), vitamin E to prevent premature bursting of red blood

AMISH FOLK MEDICINE

cells (100-800 iu).[28] Caution: excess iron stores have been shown to increase the risk for heart disease or cancer. Taking one mineral without a reasonable balance of other minerals can create a deficiency or imbalance.

BLOOD PURIFIER

The blood stream carries the "river of life" through 60,000 miles of vessels to feed all cells with nutrients and carry away waste products to be excreted through lungs, kidneys, sweat pores, or colon. The blood, not unlike a river near a major city, is often full of toxic debris. When this toxic burden becomes excessive, a little herbal help may be in order.

-Take 1/4 to 1/2 tsp. epsom salts in a 6 ounce glass of lemonade before breakfast each morning. This will cleanse the blood, kidneys, and bowels.

-Drink 8 ounces of beet juice daily.

-Chew burdock seeds to cleanse the blood and eliminate boils and styes.

-Pour one c. of boiling water over 2 T. of the following herbal concoction: 4 parts dandelion root, 4 parts burdock, 4 parts red clover, 1 part fennel seed. Let steep, cool, strain. Drink 2 T. thirty minutes after meals.

-Cleansing fast. After a 1-3 day fast (consuming water only), drink 1/4 c. unsweetened fruit or vegetable juice the first day and every 2 hours thereafter. Eating too much after a fast can be harmful and undo the benefits of the fast. You should be in good health and not diabetic to attempt a fast.

-Instead of breakfast, first thing in the morning begin sipping from a 24 ounce container of unsweetened

AMISH FOLK MEDICINE

concord grape juice. Finish the juice by 10 a.m. Eat lunch and dinner as usual, excluding any form of pork. If your stomach cannot tolerate the grape juice, then dilute it and gradually build up the concentration. Continue this grape juice semi-fast program for 6 weeks.

BLOOD IN URINE
-Drink tea from horsetail grass or comfrey root, but see a doctor first, since blood in the urine is worthy of concern.

BOILS
-Take the thin skin of the inside of a freshly broken egg shell and lay it on the sore.
-Take one tsp. of blackstrap molasses sprinkled lightly with cream of tartar, consumed twice daily.
-Drink tea from burdock.
-Dip a hydrangea leaf in boiling water and apply to the boil.
-Apply finely chopped comfrey roots to the boil.
-Mix 4 oz sublimed sulphur with 16 oz honey. Take 1 tsp. internally at bedtime.
-Make a liniment from black ointment.
-Drink red clover blossom tea.
-Make a poultice from equal parts of linseed oil (special type), honey, and flour and apply to boil.
-Consume capsules of chaparral leaves. See Poultice Section for Green Mountain Salve

BRUISES
When you bump your flesh, you may break tiny blood vessels that spill blood into the surrounding tissue and leave the recognizable blue bruise. Some people bruise far too easily, which can

AMISH FOLK MEDICINE

be an indicator of overall poor health, in particular the inability to create tough collagen (connective tissue).
-Cold wet rag applied immediately to the region will help prevent swelling and control pain.
 OTHER:
-Higher intakes of vitamin C has been shown to improve resistance to bruising. Recommendation: take 2 grams/day of vitamin C and add 1 gram each day until reaching 12 grams/day. Use buffered C if regular C causes stomach upset.
-Bioflavonoids, such as rutin and hesperidin, are accessory (helper) substances to facilitate the functions of vitamin C. Recommendation: take 200-1000 mg of rutin daily with the C.
-Another key missing ingredient in maintaining healthy connective tissue is zinc. Many Americans, particularly senior citizens, are low in zinc intake, which can lead to excessive bruising. Recommendation: take 50-100 mg/day zinc picolinate.[29]

BURNS
-For sunburn, bath in cold water.
-Apply an ice pack.
-Apply the jelly from a freshly cut aloe plant.
-Dab the burn with a cooled tea made from cheese plant (common mallow).
-Apply honey directly to the burn, cut, or sore.

AMISH FOLK MEDICINE

BURSITIS
(see also gout & rheumatism)
-Take 400-800 mg calcium supplements just as you feel the pain coming on.
-Apply vinegar to the sore area.
-Make a mixture of vinegar and water and drink to relieve bursitis.

CANCER
Cancer is basically abnormal growth that has taken over the body's normal healthy processes. Cancer can grow like a parasite, strangling vital organs, draining the body of essential nutrients, and depressing the immune system until death usually comes from infection, organ failure, or malnutrition. Cancer is a life threatening disease which requires immediate medical attention. A successful approach to the treatment of cancer would include external medicine to reduce tumor burden, coupled with stimulating the body's own internal healing mechanisms. With your doctors approval, you may want to consider some of the following therapies that augment your doctor's treatment.
-For centuries, the Amish have relied on 10-20 drops each morning of red clover to prevent cancer. Red clover is an ingredient in numerous other herbal remedies for cancer.
-For skin cancer, apply a poultice of the green flesh of the pipe organ cactus.
-For skin cancer, at night apply 1/3 grated fresh papaya bound in a sock and taped to the sore.
-For skin cancer, apply a poultice of crushed wood sorrel (oxalis) leaves.

AMISH FOLK MEDICINE

-Drink a tea from Pau d'Arco bark boiled for 10 minutes, then steeped for 10 more minutes.
-Eat 2 T. cooked asparagus daily.
-Drink a tonic made from 2 c. red clover blossoms, 1 c. berberis root (Rocky Mountain grape), 1/2 c. prickly ash root, 4 c. buckthorn, 2 c. alfalfa leaves, 1 c. pokeberry root, 1/2 c. yellow dock root. Mix herbs and fill #00 gelatin capsules. Adults take 2 capsules after each meal and at bedtime (4 times daily).
-Drink 2-3 cups daily of Jason Winters's tea. (Note: Winters developed brain cancer, then searched the world for herbal mixtures to help his otherwise untreatable condition. He now markets the herbal concoction that he feels led to his recovery.)
-Drink chapparal tea mixed with crimson clover blossoms and aloe root.
-For skin cancers, apply a poultice of dried chaparral leaves.
-For skin cancers, melt 1/2 gallon hog's lard without salt in a large kettle. Drop a large handful of fresh green rue and let it grow brown. Beat up 9 eggs and add. When the mixture turns brown, discard the herbs and cool. Apply topically to suspicious areas.

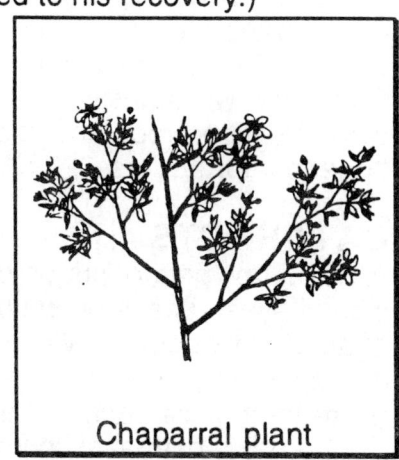

Chaparral plant

-Boil 1 lb fresh figs slowly in 1 gallon fresh cow's milk until figs are soft. Remove figs from mixture and stir in a separate container until figs develop poultice texture. Every 12 hours, apply a poultice of the figs

AMISH FOLK MEDICINE

and drink 1 c. of the remaining milk solution. Skin cancer should break open in 24-48 hours and then begin healing.

-Start by taking 1 drop of USP (United States Pharmacopoeia) iodine in a half glass of water after each meal. The second day, take 2 drops per dose. Each day add 1 extra drop until you have a warm or queer feeling in your stomach. Decrease the dose until you feel comfortable again. Continue this regimen.

-Create herbal concoction consisting of: 1 c. bloodroot, 2 c. red clover blossoms, 1 T. ginger. Add 1 quart of water and boil down to 1 pint. Strain and add 1 pint of whiskey. Take 1 tsp. 3 times/day.

-Many generations have used salves to treat skin cancer. One formula commercially available is Cansema, which includes a proprietary blend of zinc chloride, blood root, and chaparral. See sources in appendix for address.

CATARACTS

-Scrape raw potato, put on cloth, and apply to the closed eyes. Leave on overnight. Or, press juice out of an old raw potato. With an eye dropper put two drops into each eye every evening before retiring. Make fresh juice each evening.

-Twice daily, bath eyes in warm salt water followed by warm vinegar water.

OTHER:

-Numerous clinicians are reporting reversal of cataracts with supplements that include high dose antioxidants: 800 iu vitamin E, 5 grams vitamin C, 15,000 iu beta-carotene, plus 30 mg zinc.[30]

AMISH FOLK MEDICINE

-There is also good evidence that a diet low in calories, sugar, and dairy products coupled with optimal levels of various vitamins and minerals can prevent or delay the onset of cataracts.[31]

CIRCULATION
-To improve circulation and warmth, soak feet in hot water with a bit of red pepper.
-Use inner soles in the shoes made of wool felt to keep feet warm.
-Drink a weak tea made from the leaves and flowers of the hawthorne berry (crataegus oxycantha).
-Eat cayenne peppers or fill small capsules with cayenne powder and take twice daily with plenty of fluid.
-Boil a one inch section of bloodroot in 1 c. of water for a few minutes. Take 1 T. each day.
-Drink tansy tea 3-4 times daily.

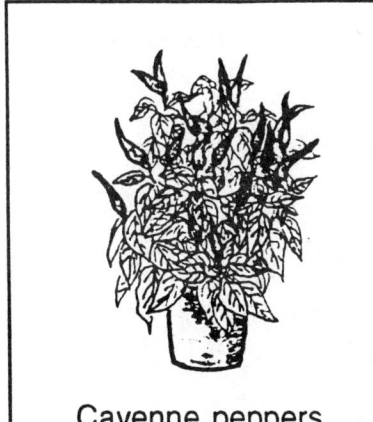

Cayenne peppers

COLDS
-Take vitamins A & D throughout the winter to prevent colds.
-To warm the throat and make a hostile environment for the germs, gargle with hot salt water, spit it out. Repeat in 15 minutes.
-To both prevent and help cure colds, cut open a fresh onion and lay it out on the kitchen shelf.
-Boil a pot of water with peppermint oil or pine oil so the house occupants will inhale the vapors.

AMISH FOLK MEDICINE

-Rub the outside of the throat glands with camphor or Vicks, then cover with flannel cloth.
-Drink lots of herbal teas, unsweetened juices, lemon tea, or hot chicken broth.
-Place a drop of peppermint oil in a bowl of boiling water with the face held close to inhale the vapors.
-Place a drop of peppermint oil in a tsp. of brown sugar and swallow.
-Place a drop of peppermint oil on a handkerchief and place to the nose before retiring in the evening.
-For children, place a drop of peppermint oil on their pillowcase at night before sleeping.
-Drink sage tea.
-Give children (over 2 years) a tsp. of honey before putting them to bed to help them breath easier.
-Place a drop of salt water solution (8 ounces water with 1/2 tsp. salt) in the nostrils, or use nasal purge as described in "allergy" section.
-Take 1 T. daily of cod liver oil to build resistance.
-To break a fever, juice 1/2 lemon, fill a glass with water, add 1/2 tsp. of bicarbonate of soda. Drink this solution every half hour until fever breaks.
-Drink hot lemon tea with honey. Juice 1/2 lemon for each cup of tea.
-When first symptoms of flu appear, take 1 tsp. of vinegar, a sprinkle of bicarbonate of soda, red pepper, and ginger in 1/2 c. of warm water.
-Boil 1 gallon of dandelion flowers in 1 gallon of water for 5 minutes. Let stand for 3 days in a glass jug or stainless steel container. Strain, then boil the peelings of 2 lemons and 1 orange in the dandelion water for 15 minutes. Let stand until lukewarm. Slice in the 2 lemons and 1 orange. Add 2 tsp. yeast and 3 lb. sugar. Cover with cloth and let stand 6 days.

AMISH FOLK MEDICINE

Bottle. When having a cold, take 1 T. at bedtime or as needed.
OTHER:
-High doses of vitamin C have been shown to lower the incidence, duration, and severity of colds.[32] Recommendation: take 1-5 grams of vitamin C daily, and 1 gram/hour if you have a cold.
-Zinc lozenges have been shown to reduce the duration and intensity of a cold.[33] Recommendations: Take 1 zinc lozenge (15 mg. zinc) every 3 hours while having a cold.

COLD SORES

Herpes simplex is a nasty virus that seems to permanently reside in certain unfortunate individuals. It is spread by mucus in people who are genetically vulnerable. It flares up in times of emotional or physical stress.
-Drink sage tea.
OTHER:
-Vitamin C supplements (1-2 grams) virtually eliminated flareups in 30 of 38 cold sore patients.[34]
-Bioflavonoid supplements (1000-1500 mg) helped 2/3 of herpes subjects.[35]
-Topical vitamin E provided pain relief for herpes sores.[36]
-L-lysine (1-6 grams) tripled the recovery rate for herpes patients.[37]

COLIC

-Make a tea by boiling 1 c. water with 1 tsp. fennel seeds. Cool to lukewarm, strain.
-Prepare a tea from chamomile and/or catnip.

AMISH FOLK MEDICINE

-Give peppermint or spearmint tea.
-To remove sour vomit odor, fill a container with baking soda and place in room.
   OTHER:
-If the nursing mother discontinues eating dairy products (milk, cheese, ice cream, etc.), then she may see a dramatic improvement in her child's colic. The child's allergy to cow's milk is caused by mother's consumption of milk products.
-Change formula from cow's milk to goat milk, which is closer in nutrient content to human milk.

COLON PROBLEMS
(constipation, colitis)

-Eat more roughage, which includes unprocessed fruits, vegetables, whole grains, and beans. A favorite Amish cereal recipe: 6 cups oatmeal, 1 c. shredded coconut, 3 c. wheat germ, 1/2 c. chopped almonds, 1/2 c. chopped pecans, 1.5 c. brown sugar, 1/2 tsp. salt, 1/2 c. vegetable oil. Mix in big bowl then toast until crunchy.
-Teas made from senna leaf, or flaxseed, or psyllium seed help.
-Chew well then swallow 1 tsp. flaxseed.
-Take magnesium supplements (400 mg. daily) or take 1 tsp. epsom salts with glass of warm water.
-Get more exercise, which helps the muscles of the abdomen move the food to the colon.
-May be caused by too many gravies, pastries, breads, and not enough exercise.
-Avoid white flour and fried foods.
-Drink at least 6 glasses daily of purified water. Sprinkle in some powdered vitamin C to neutralize cancer-causing nitrates in the stomach.

AMISH FOLK MEDICINE

-Sprinkle 1 tsp. ground flaxseed on your cereal each morning. Or boil the flax seeds then strain and drink the tea.
-For lower bowel problems, use enema of either 8 ounces lukewarm black coffee, or warm salt water solution (8 ounces water with 1/2 tsp. sea salt).
-Boil flax seeds in water, strain, then drink the tea.
-Drink a glass of hot water on rising in the morning.
-Skip a meal or two, then drink unsweetened juices for a half a day or longer.
-Give your organs a rest by eating less. Eat plenty of raw salads and fruits.
-Take 1 tsp. ground psyllium seeds in 1/2 c. unsweetened juice in the morning upon arising and in the evening. In the morning follow with a large capsule filled with epsom salts. Continue for 2 weeks.
-To make your own suppositories, mix 1 oz. each of goldenseal, boric acid, white flour in with glycerine until stiff. Form into suppositories and refrigerate. When needed, insert in rectum at bedtime and leave until morning.
-Consume only unlimited amounts of grape juice for 3 days.
-Take 1 tsp. powdered psyllium seed with fruit juice about 15 minutes before breakfast.
-Put one rounded tsp. of slippery elm powder into a glass with hot milk. This may be used on cereal. Follow this procedure in the evening and every day until relieved. Psyllium seed cleanses the colon and slippery elm aids healing.
-Drink 1-2 c. golden seal tea. Take a gulp every few hours during the day for 2 weeks. Quit a few days occasionally, then continue.

AMISH FOLK MEDICINE

-Drink a quart of peppermint tea daily, sweetened with honey.
-Use enemas with warm water tea made from burdock roots or inner white oak bark. Use 2 T. of root or bark to 1.5 quarts of water. Let brew, then cool to desired temperature. Strain through cloth. Take one high enema daily for 6 days, then only occasionally as needed.
-Make a drink from 1/4 tsp. powdered myrrh and 1/4 tsp. golden seal in 1/2 glass of very warm water. Also take 5 grams of garlic capsules 3 times/day.
-Avoid cold water, sugar, pastries, onions, black pepper, and pickled foods.
-Olive oil, prune juice, buttermilk, or yogurt in the diet will prevent and treat constipation.
-To relieve diarrhea of colitis: boil wild blackberry root or red oak bark in water and drink 1/2 c. If not relieved drink another 1/2 c. in several hours.
-Take 1 T. of safflower oil each day to heal the lining of the colon.
-Take 1 T. of flaxseed oil (dietary linseed oil) to speed healing of the colon.
-For piles, drink a tea from sumac tops before bedtime and upon arising; or apply a poultice of jimson weeds fried in lard and spread on area.
-For relief from piles, steam the affected part by sitting over a pan containing garlic boiled in milk.
   OTHER:
-Many diseases are precipitated by constipation. Regularity is a hallmark of a healthy body. Typically, a diet high in fiber (food from plants) and water will provide excellent regularity for most individuals. Some people may need to add supplements of fiber to encourage daily bowel movements. Laxatives and

AMISH FOLK MEDICINE

enemas should be used sparingly, as they can be habit forming and make the bowels lazy.
-Assist the muscles of the intestines by stomach massaging. Do this by using the palm side of a closed fist to rock gently over the intestinal area. This helps to move the fecal matter through the intestines for elimination.
-An excellent laxative is high doses of vitamin C. Many experts feel that the ideal intake of vitamin C is just below "bowel tolerance", or the level which causes diarrhea. For most healthy adults, this "bowel tolerance" is in the range of 10-20 grams/day. The high doses of C provide many benefits in the system, while helping to encourage regularity in the bowels.[38]

CORNS

-Soak a small piece of cloth in vinegar. Bind it on the toe, leaving it on day and night. The corn will come out by the root.
-For corns, soak feet in warm water for 15 minutes, then apply the inside of a small piece of lemon peel to the corn and tape it there overnight. After three nights, the corn should lift out.

COUGH

-Mix equal parts of lemon juice, honey, and castor oil. Adults take 1T./day and children over 2 yrs. old take 1tsp/day.
-Steep 1/2 tsp. dried crushed green peach tree leaves in 1 quart boiling water for 10 minutes. Take 1 T. of this tea every hour with a few drops of honey.
-Steep 4 chestnut leaves in 1 pint boiling water. Sweeten with honey and drink 5-6 times daily.

AMISH FOLK MEDICINE

-Boil one lemon, squeeze out the juice, add 1 c. honey. Take 1-2 T. at bedtime or as needed.
-Drink fenugreek tea to eliminate mucus.
-Make a cough syrup by washing mullein leaves, boil for 10 minutes, add enough sugar for flavor, then boil down to a thick syrup.
-Use vinegar as a gargle to help clear up a cough.
-Gargle with hot salt water or hot sumac tea.
-Drink a tea made from slippery elm bark and horehound.
-Peel and slice onions. Fry them until brown. Place these tolerably warm onions between two large clean washcloths or handkerchiefs and lay on the chest for a poultice.
-Apply Po Ho oil to chest.
-To make cough drops, mix 1 oz. cubeb powder, 2 oz. gum arabic, 2 oz. licorice root powdered, and 1 lb. powdered sugar with 4 T. water.
-To make a cough syrup, mix 8 oz. of honey with 7 drops of eucalyptus oil (or cherry bark) and stir well. Take a few drops when needed.
-To make a cough syrup, cut 1 lb. of fresh garlic into slices. Add garlic to 1 quart boiling water in jar, cover, and let stand for 12 hours. Boil 1 tsp. each of: bruised caraway and fennel seeds in 4 oz. vinegar; then strain and add to garlic mixture. Add honey for flavor and give 1-2 T. when needed.
-Rub the chest, back, and throat with goose fat.
-A swallow of pineapple juice on regular basis helps.
-Mix 2 T. brown sugar, 1 T. butter, 2 T. vinegar. Heat until melted. Blend. While still warm, serve 1 tsp. to patient.
-Inhale the warm vapors from a bath or shower of hot water. Loosens the mucus in the throat and lungs.

AMISH FOLK MEDICINE

-Steep 1/3 c. hoarhound with 1 tsp. sassafras in 1 quart boiling water for 10-15 minutes. Strain, then add 1/4 c. honey. Take a swallow or two when bothered.
-Put an ounce lobelia in a pint of boiling water. Cool. Take 2 T. every 4 hours.
-Mix 1/4 oz. lobelia, black cohosh root, and chestnut leaves in a jar. Pour 1/2 pint boiling water on the herbs and let stand for 30 minutes. Strain, then add 1 lb. sugar and bring to a boil. Remove scum and give 1 tsp. every hour to children.
-Simmer one thinly sliced lemon and 1/2 pint flaxseed in 1 quart water for 4 hours. Strain while hot. Add 2 oz. honey. Take 1 T. three times daily or more after severe coughing session.

CRAMPS

-For a "charley horse", drink at least a quart of milk/day.
-Eat 4-8 soda crackers/day.
-Drink 1 tsp. of vinegar/day.
-Rub olive oil on the sole of the foot.
-Soak the feet in hot water.
-For general cramps, drink a hot tea made with 1/4 tsp. ginger.
-Drink a hot tea made with thyme.
-For monthly female cramps, make a poultice from catnip and rub on the abdomen.

DEODORANT

-Mix 1 T. vegetable oil, 2 T. cornstarch, 2 T. bicarbonate of soda in a small pan heated on stove until blended. Store in small container and apply as deodorant.

AMISH FOLK MEDICINE

OTHER:
-The body's odor is reflective of what is happening inside. Strong foul odors from the skin indicates illness, poor diet, or toxin buildup.
-Easiest way to eliminate body odor is to eliminate the place that most bacteria can buildup: shave the hairs in the armpit. You will not need deodorant.
-Realize that many deodorants either block pores to reduce the outlets for poisons, or worse yet some contain aluminum which can be absorbed by the skin and buildup into Alzheimer's disease.
-Eat less fat and less red meat for a sweeter smell.
-Sweat at least once each day, preferably by exercise, but also by hot showers and tubs to keep the skin pores flushed out. There are 3500 sweat pores per postage-stamp-sized space on your skin. Altogether, you have 40 miles of pores that need to be flushed and drained often.

DIABETES
In addition to following your doctor's directions, you may want to consider the following:
-Drink 3 cups daily of tea from boiling 1/4 avocado leaf, 1 eucalyptus leaf, and 1 walnut leaf.
-Drink a tea from peach leaf (1 leaf per c.).
-Drink a tea from marshmallow (cheese plant).
-Take capsules containing the following combination: cedar berries, uva ursi, licorice root, mullein, cayenne, and golden seal root.
-Drink tea from strawberry leaf or Pau d'Arco to lower blood sugar levels.
-Drink tea from arrowbruce or blueberry leaf to stimulate pancreatic health.

AMISH FOLK MEDICINE

-Eat artichokes like apples.
-Kelp (seaweed, or sea vegetables) in the diet often helps.
-Plenty of oatmeal and dried beans help the diabetic.
-Drink tea made from clover blossoms and dandelions.
-Drink tea made from cheese plant (kas bobbla).
   OTHER:
-There is plenty of scientific evidence showing that most diabetics can be helped through nutrition, while some can be "cured". Reduce body fat. Eat less refined carbohydrates, including white sugar and white flour. Take daily supplements of chromium picolinate (400-600 mcg), carnitine (1-2 grams), B-6 (50-100 mg), vitamin E (2,000 iu), zinc (30-50 mg), inositol ("muscle sugar" 1-2 grams), ginseng (500 mg), and eat fenugreek (a leguminous plant) often.[39]

DIAPER RASH
-Apply vitamin E ointment to trouble area.
-Rub vaseline over the entire diaper area before putting the baby to bed in the evening.
-For prickly heat, rub the affected parts with the inside of watermelon rind. Or sponge with equal parts of water and vinegar.
-Apply ointment containing vitamins A & D.
-Be sure to dry diapers in sunlight after washing them to eliminate fungus.
-Apply cornstarch when changing diapers.

DIARRHEA
-Drink tea made from caraway seeds.
-Eat 1/2 c. blueberries.

AMISH FOLK MEDICINE

-Brew tea from either: slippery elm, or blackberry, or dried blackberry roots, or red raspberry leaf, or white oak bark.
-Drink tea made from leaves of green soupbean plant.
-Bring 1 c. of milk to a boil. Add 1 tsp. nutmet, 1/8 tsp. cinnamon, and honey. Drink at mealtime instead of eating heavy food.
-Mix 1 tsp. flour with 1 tsp. nutmeg, 1 tsp. white sugar, and pinch of salt in glass. Add enough water to make easy to drink. Take every 4 hours.
-For children, give 2 tsp. vinegar every 2 hours.
-Boil carrots, then puree. Take 1 tsp. every 15 minutes.
-Cook rice until soft. For infants, give rice water with a bit of sugar and milk. For older children, eat the whole rice.
-Mix 1/2 c. fresh orange juice, 1 T. sugar, 1/6 tsp. salt, 1 1/3 c water. Give child 1/2 ounce of this every 2 hours.
-Summertime diarrhea may be brought on by drinking too much cold fluids.
-Drink boneset tea.
-Mix 1/2 oz each of scullcap, feverfew, and lady slipper. Place in quart jar, then fill with boiling water, let steep for 2 hours. Take 2 T. three times daily.
-Drink tea from black snake grass roots.

DIGESTION & STOMACH PROBLEMS
-To purge the body of amoebic parasites, make a tea from 1 tsp. mango tree bark in 1 c. boiling water.
-To purge the body of parasites, eat 1 papaya leaf daily or take 3-6 garlic capsules daily.

AMISH FOLK MEDICINE

-To rid the body of worms, mix this anti-parasite syrup: fennel seed, black walnut hulls, senna leaves, male fern, tansey, tame sage, and wormwood.
-Drink a tea from pumpkin seeds to rid the body of parasites.

DROPSY (edema, fluid retention)
-Boil 6 one inch pieces of Christ root in 2 c. water for 5 minutes. Take 1 T. several times daily.
-Drink a tea of horsetail grass, stinging nettle, rosemary, and birch leaves.
-Mix 1 gallon pure apple cider, 1 handful of horseradish, 2 handfuls of parsley, 2 T. mustard seeds, 1 ounce juniper berries. Let stand in a warm place for 24 hours, strain, then drink 2 T. 4-5 times daily.

In children...
EARACHE (or if persists see a doctor)
-Use fresh sheep wool with lanolin still intact. Make a wad and put in ears.
-Place a cold wet washrag on ears.
-To relieve pain, dip cotton wad in molasses and stuff into ears.
-Add a few drops of Oil of Herbs to the ears.
-Use otagesine, product available in health food stores.
-Mix 1 T. each olive oil with oil of rue and place several drops in the ears.
-Rub olive oil, or herb oil, or Vicks on the area surrounding the ears.
-Gather small mullein (wool draut) flowers. Put them in a bottle and place in the sun. The flowers emit an oil. Put 1-2 drops of the oil in the ears then plug with cotton.

AMISH FOLK MEDICINE

ECZEMA
-Apply a paste made from lard and sulphur to the affected region. Make sure to wear old clothes over the sulphur-lard, since this ruins clothes.
-Eat 2 T. brewer's yeast daily.
-Apply vitamin E liquid to the affected skin.
-Apply a salve of emulsified fish oil to the skin. Cover with flannel and tape on.
-Drink goat's milk.

ENDURANCE, ENERGY
(see also "tonic")
-Mix 1 T. each of finely chopped yellow dock, burdock, dandelion, black snake root, and sassafras bark into a jar of wine and let stand for 3 months. Take one T. each morning before breakfast.
-Drink tansy tea often.
-Soak 1 T. chia seeds overnight in a c. of water, strain, and drink liquid in the morning.
-An afternoon nap of 30 minutes is equal in sleep value to 2 hours at night.

EYES
-Drink tea made from eyebright or goldenseal herbs.
-To improve eye health, take 6-10 capsules daily of carrot seed oil.
-Growth of cataracts can be retarded by adding 1 drop of flaxseed oil in eyes at bedtime.
-Use elderberry blossom tea as an eye wash to cure pink eye.
-Warm chamomile tea dropped into eyes will cure styes.

AMISH FOLK MEDICINE

-If you have a tiny irritant in the eye, then put a single flaxseed under the eyelid. The irritant will be drawn to the seed, which should be removed shortly.

FEMALE PROBLEMS
(Menopause: change of life)
-Drinking a tea made from chestnut leaves was known to be good for this trouble.
-Create a herbal tea concoction from rosemary, horsetail, grass, yarrow, shepherd's purse, dwarf elder, peppermint. Drink 2 cups/day, with a swallow now and again.
    OTHER:
-A female gynecologist has found tremendous success with her clients by giving 2,000 iu/day vitamin E to relieve hot flashes.[40]

FERTILITY
-For both men and women, consume 1 T. daily of both carrot seed oil and wheat germ oil.
-Eat a diet rich in alfalfa sprouts.
-Abstain from working around pesticides and other questionable chemicals.
-Men should avoid wearing tights pants and heavy cotton underwear as this added warmth cuts down on sperm count.
-Pumpkin seeds or 50 mg/day of zinc supplements can help men.
    OTHER:
-Excellent studies show that fertility in women can be improved by: maintaining proper weight, avoiding caffeine and alcohol, taking supplements of B-6 (100-300 mg). Fertility for men can be improved by: avoiding alcohol, taking B-12 (6000 mcg), vitamin C

AMISH FOLK MEDICINE

(1-2 grams), zinc (30-60 mg), and L-arginine (4 grams).[41]

FEVER
-Make a paste with flour and vinegar. Spread on a cloth and apply to the bottom of the patient's feet.
-Beat one egg white with 1 tsp. sugar and 1/4 c. water. Drink this solution.
-Make tea from the bark of weeping willow tree. Simmer for 5 minutes. Add willow leaves, then steep for at least 15 minutes. Take 1 tsp. of this tea washed down with 1 c. water. Dilute more for children.
-Drink tea from pennyroyal, lobelia, or red clover (1/2 tsp. per c. water).
-Drink tea from strawberry leaf, or alfalfa, or yarrow.

FISHBONE STUCK IN THROAT
- After calling 911:

-Gargle with vinegar or take a few swallows of strong vinegar, which may soften the bones.
-Break an egg into a glass and have them swallow it.
   OTHER:
-Try to dislodge obstruction by thumping on back or turning upside down, or grabbing around waist just below the rib cage and forcefully squeezing.

FROSTBITE
-Mix 1 oz. each of olive oil, peppermint oil, and ammonia and rub on frostbitten hands.
-Soak frostbitten hands in cold water. Rub hands but do not hold directly to heat.

FLU (see also "cold")
-To relieve chest congestion, mix a salve of 6 oz. sheep tallow, 15 oz. valeine, 3 oz. menthol crystals, 3

AMISH FOLK MEDICINE

oz. beeswax; then melt and add 2 oz. gum camphor oil, 2 oz. sassafras oil, 2 oz. eucalyptus oil. Apply this mixture liberally to the chest.

-Special remedy for children: make a large pot of tea from Queen Anne's lace and use this for a hot foot bath for children while draping their body with warm wool blankets. At the same time, have the children drink elder blossom tea.

-Drink a tea from elderberry flowers.

-Drink a tea from 1/4 tsp. cayenne in 1 c. hot water. Encourages the body to sweat.

-Drink a tea from equal parts bayberry bark, ginger root, cloves, cayenne, and white pine bark.

-Drink a tea from 1 lb. bayberry bark, 1 lb. ginger root, 2 oz. cayenne pepper, 2 oz. cloves. Finely pulverize and mix ingredients. Mix 1/4 tsp. of herbal concoction with 1 tsp. sugar in a cup of boiling water. Let stand and drink.

GALLBLADDER & GALLSTONES

-Take 1 tsp. parsley juice every morning upon arising.

-Take the juice of 1-2 lemons before retiring at night. Drink undiluted, then lie on right side for 20 minutes.

-Juice 3 lemons, add 3 tsp. cream of tartar, 3 tsp. epsom salts. Put in pint jar of water. Take 1 T. of this solution each morning before breakfast.

-Take 1 tsp. olive oil followed immediately by 1 tsp. lemon juice. Do this three times daily for 3 consecutive days while fasting.

-Drink a solution of 6 oz. olive oil with 6 oz. pure lemon juice to eliminate gallstones.

-For gallstones, drink a gallon of pure apple juice for two consecutive days, averaging 1 c./hour. Fast for

AMISH FOLK MEDICINE

these 2 days. On the third morning, begin with drinking 4 oz. pure cold pressed olive oil. Gradually return to solid foods. May also help kidney stones.
-Eat nothing but grapefruit or grapefruit juice until relieved.
-Before retiring, take 6 oz olive oil with a bit of water. First thing in the morning, take 1 tsp. epsom salts with some water.
-Make a tea from 10 tsp. ground root of sweet weed and 1/2 tsp. sacred bark boiled in 1 pint of water for 1 hour. Strain through cheesecloth and cool. Consume 1/2 c. daily until relief comes.

GAS (flatulence)
-Swallow 2 capsules daily of ginger root, or drink hot ginger tea, or homemade ginger ale.
-Chew 1 tsp. of coriander seeds or caraway seeds.
-Drink warm mint tea with meals.
-Eat slowly. Food consumed quickly has many trapped pockets of gas.
-Avoid carbonated drinks, like soda pop.
-Mix the following herbs and take capsules at dinner time: fennel, wild yam, catnip, ginger, peppermint, spearmint, papaya, and lobelia.

GOUT
-Apply a poultice of chopped fresh onions daily.
-Eat a diet with 2 cups fresh cherries and no meat.
-Take capsules with yucca and devil's claw leaves.

HAIR & SKIN CARE
HAIR:
-Use Vel bar soap (or castile soap) to shampoo hair and vinegar to rinse the hair.

AMISH FOLK MEDICINE

-Beat egg whites and apply to the scalp. Let stand for 3 minutes. Rinse well.
-Add several drops of baby oil (mineral oil) to the hair rinse solution for better managed hair.
-Shampoo with a mixture of rosemary leaves, chamomile leaves, rosewater, and mild soap. Can add 1 beaten egg with natural coconut oil to this mixture.

BALDNESS:

-For baldness, consume 40 drops daily of red clover tops liquid extract. Use a scalp rinse of vinegar with sage tea.
-Take 30-60 mg supplemental zinc daily.
-Rub aloe vera into the scalp for thinning hair.

DANDRUFF:

-Rub a small amount of pure coconut oil in the scalp daily.
-Use tea from burdock or sage as a scalp rinse after shampoo.
-Dissolve 1 tsp. borax (boric acid) in 1 c. water. Using a brush, wet the hair with this solution every day for a week, then twice each week for 3 weeks.
-Mix 1/2 oz sulphur in a pint of water. Let stand for 2 days while shaking occasionally. Dampen the scalp 3-4 times/week with this solution.
-Gather stinging nettles with gloves on. Boil 1 c stinging nettles in 1 pint of water and add 1 T vinegar. Cool and strain. Use this tea for rinsing the hair.

SKIN:

-Mix 1/4 c. olive oil with 1 tsp. sugar and massage hands twice weekly with solution.

AMISH FOLK MEDICINE

-Mix 1 oz glycerine, 1 oz rubbing alcohol, 1 oz camphor spirit, 1 oz of 10% ammonia and use this solution for a hand creme.

-For a lotion to heal dry skin, mix 4 oz. glycerine, 4 oz. alcohol, 1 oz. quince seed. First pour one pint boiling water on quince seed and let soak overnight, then strain and add other ingredients.

-Apply a mixture of equal parts bay rum and glycerine.

-Make a paste of cornstarch and evaporated milk. Apply to face and throat. Let dry. Bath with cold water to remove.

-For dry skin, mix together a salve of equal parts of cocoa butter, glycerine, lanolin, rosewater, and elderflower water.

-For eczema, gather black poplar buds (balm of Gilead) in the spring when buds are sticky, boil in olive oil, strain, make a salve.

-Make herbal capsules from equal parts barberry, wild yam, cramp bark, fennel seed, ginger, catnip, and peppermint. Take 2 capsules 15 minutes before bedtime.

-For white spots on skin, make a salve of hog lard, limes, and sulphur.

SCAR TISSUE:

-To help prevent scar tissue from forming, repeatedly rub cocoa butter on wound.

-To help prevent scarring, apply vitamin E ointment to wound.

-To help dissolve scar tissue, rub on castor oil

FRECKLING:

-To reduce freckling, bathe the face in fresh buttermilk. Or mix 2 oz. sour milk with 2 drams grated horseradish, 6 drams cornmeal; spread this mixture

AMISH FOLK MEDICINE

between thin muslin and apply to affected parts at night, making sure not to get into eyes.

HEADACHE
-Often caused by stress. Learn the art of relaxation.
-Take 1/4 tsp. soda in a c. of warm water before going to bed and upon arising.
-Using forefinger pressure, massage the back of the neck.
-Saturate a cloth in ice cold vinegar, squeeze out excess, then bind around forehead.
-Soak feet for 10-20 minutes in a hot foot bath to which 2 tsp. powdered mustard has been added. At the same time, apply to the forehead a handkerchief well dampened with equal parts of water and vinegar.
-Apply a lotion of oil of rosemary at the temples and gently massage in to skin, keeping away from the eyes.
   OTHER:
-The herb feverfew has been demonstrated effective in the treatment of migraine headaches.[42]

HEART & BLOOD PRESSURE
-For irregular heart beat mix 1 tsp. each of black cohosh, scullcap, valerian, lobelia, and cayenne in 1 pint of boiling water. Drink 1-2 cups of this tea daily.
-The Amish eat an apple a day to keep the doctor away, and plenty of garlic each day to keep everybody else away!
-Vitamin E, C, and lecithin are advised for the heart. Many Amish men take 100-300 iu daily of vitamin E. Whole wheat bread can add substantially to vitamin E intake.

AMISH FOLK MEDICINE

-Avoid excess of high cholesterol foods, including eggs, bacon, ham, butter, cheese, ice cream, milk (except for children), and chocolate.
-Daily consume a tea made from Hawthorn berries and cayenne (red pepper).
-Teas made from sassafras, burdock, or red clover help to thin and cleanse the blood.
-Exercise helps to prevent heart attacks. Walk daily. A mini-trampoline in the home can be helpful.
-Teas from rosemary, chamomile, or red pepper before retiring each night help to improve circulation.
-Phlebitis (inflammation of the veins) can be relieved by taking 1 tsp. safflower oil before breakfast, 3 garlic oil capsules before meals, 3 cups alfalfa seed tea daily (2 tsp. crushed seeds in 1 c. boiling water). Also, to relieve the pain of phlebitis, apply a salve of ginseng, aloe vera, allantoin, vitamins A, D, E, and B-6.
-Palpitations of the heart can be caused by gas upset in the stomach, which can be relieved by drinking 8 oz water with 1/2 tsp. bicarbonate of soda.
-Ten minutes before breakfast, mix 1 T. honey with 3 tsp. vinegar in 8 oz. warm water and drink.
-For high blood pressure, mix 1/2 tsp. cream of tartar, 2 T. sulphur, and 2 T. epsom salts in 1 quart water. Shake well and take 2 T. daily.
-Garlic, lecithin, and asparagus help control blood pressure.
-Mix 2 tsp. cider vinegar with 1 tsp. honey in 8 oz water and drink 10 minutes before bedtime.
-Avoid lard, fatty foods, margarine, shortening, and peanuts. Or eat nothing but unsweetened fruit for 2 days.

AMISH FOLK MEDICINE

-Sesame seeds help to prevent fatty buildup in the arteries. Make a useful candy by mixing sesame seeds with a small amount of honey, form into balls, and keep in freezer.

OTHER:

-In a 17 year study of thousands of people, researchers found that the most important nutritional predictor of heart disease was the amount of vitamin E in the blood. Vitamin E helps to prevent the "rusting" of fats, which eventually block the arteries and lead to heart disease. A diet high in fiber, green and orange vegetables, and whole grains will lower the risk for heart disease. Daily supplements of: vitamin E (300-800 iu), vitamin C (1-5 grams), garlic (6 capsules), fish oil (1 T. oil), and chromium picolinate (400 mcg) will dramatically lower the risk for, and, in some cases, even reverse heart disease.[43]

HEMORRHOIDS & PILES

-To a hot sitz bath, add 1 lb. alum.
-Apply a poultice from marigold, malva, comfrey, red clover, burdock, elder, and yellow dock.
-May be caused by eating too much grapefruit.
-Omit pork from the diet for relief.
-Eat raw red beets between meals.

OTHER:

-Use toilet paper soaked in warm water to cleanse yourself, then dry toilet paper to dry yourself. This method alone virtually eliminates hemorrhoid pain in most people. Keep a cup of water by the toilet, or bring a warmed cup of water with you into the bathroom.

AMISH FOLK MEDICINE

HICCUPS
-Take a few rapid swallows of canned pineapple juice. Repeat each hour if necessary.
-Just drinking water may help.
-Add 1/3 tsp. cream of tartar to 8 oz. warm water. Drink 2 T. at a time on empty stomach.
-Eat 1 tsp. peanut butter.
-Drink the juice from 1/2 orange.
-Hold the breath as long as you can.
-Take a tsp. of honey.
   OTHER:
-Place a paper bag over your head, crimping the bag around the neck with your hands but allowing circulation in the throat region. Breath 4-5 times in a relaxed even method, then remove bag. Using the bag helps to equalize the ratio between carbon dioxide (exhaled) and oxygen (inhaled) in the bloodstream.

HIVES
-Each morning drink a blend of 1/2 tsp. soda, 1/2 tsp. tartar, and 1 tsp. epsom salts in 4 oz water.
-Steep catnip leaves in boiling water for 10 minutes. Strain, then wash the hives with the solution.

INGROWN TOENAIL
-Do not trim too far down on the sides of the toenail.
-Put peroxide on sore spot to cleanse.
-Soak the feet at least once daily in hot water.
-Cut a V-shape out of the front center of the toenail to find relief from toenail pain.

INSECT BITES & BEE STINGS

AMISH FOLK MEDICINE

-Make a poultice paste of equal parts bicarbonate of soda and vinegar.
-Apply a fresh cut onion to the sting.
-Make a poultice by mixing 2 oz. olive oil, 1 dram carbolic acid, 1 dram pennyroyal, 1 dram cedar oil, 2 drams citronella oil, 2 drams tincture of camphor, and 1/2 dram acetic acid. Apply to bites to lessen sting, or as an insect repellant.
-To relieve itching, moisten a bar of soap and rub it on the sting.
-As an insect repellant, apply citronella on skin. Helps pets, too.
-Remove the stinger by laying a paring knife flat against the skin, sliding the sharp edge against the skin to draw it out. Do not try to pick it out with the fingers as this will only spread the poison. Once stinger is out, then bruise a plantain and rub into the sting.
-Dissolve 1/4 tsp. meat tenderizer in 1 tsp. water and rub into the skin around the sting.
-To keep insects away, keep an infusion of chamomile flowers in a bottle throughout the summertime and apply to the skin before going outdoors.
-To ease pain, rub one of the following on the sting: raw potato, lemon slice, poppy leaves, marigold, or nasturtium leaves.
-Make a poultice of ground saffron tea and apply to the sting.
-Apply a slice of raw onion to the sting.
-Apply a poultice of baking soda and water to the sting.
    OTHER:

AMISH FOLK MEDICINE

-Make a poultice from chewing tobacco or shredded cigars with warm water. Form a thick paste. Apply to the insect sting. Has been known to even reverse allergic reactions to stings.
-Electrical energy tends to neutralize or "denature" the poisonous proteins from stings and bites. For particularly dangerous snake and spider bites, use an electric "stun gun" to the injured area with electrodes on either side of the bite. Not for small children, but has been known to neutralize potentially lethal bites.

INSOMNIA
-Cultivate beautiful thoughts, especially in the evening. Listen to music or read poetry.
-Soak 1 tsp. plain gelatin in 1 c. boiling water then stir until mixed. Take 2 tsp. of this drink at supper time.
-Near bedtime, soak feet in hot water with 1/4 c. vinegar added.
-The following herbs in capsule or tea form may help: hops, vervain, valerian, scullcap, catnip, peppermint, and golden seal.
-Take 1-2 tsp. honey before retiring.
-Drink a glass of warm milk before bedtime.
-Many a mother has given catnip tea to babies to help them rest.
    OTHER:
-In scientific studies on humans, valerian has been shown to improve sleep patterns without inducing any "hangover" effect.[44]

ITCHING

AMISH FOLK MEDICINE

-Cover the itch with a poultice of cornstarch and let it dry on the skin.
-Apply witch hazel or rubbing alcohol.
-Add 1 tsp. soda to 1 quart of water and wash itch area.
-Place 3 cups cooked oatmeal in a cheesecloth bag and soak in warm water for 15 minutes. Then use bag to rub over itch.

KIDNEY & BLADDER
-Drink teas made from one or more of the following: nettle, yarrow (schaf ribbe), broom grass (gravel grass), burdock (gletta), dandelion root, and golden seal. Dried and roasted dandelion root can be used as a coffee substitute.
-To reduce fluid retention, drink tea made from corn silk.
-To help pass kidney stones, drink cucumber juice.
-To help in kidney stones, drink tea from 1/2 avocado leaf.
-For kidney problems, steep 3 tsp. brown corn seed in a pint of water and drink 1 c. daily.
-To help painlessly pass a kidney stone, eat no food but consume large amounts of unsweetened apple juice.
-Make a tea from 3 avocado leaves in one c. boiling water, steeped for 10 minutes.
-Vinegar tea or cranberry juice may help some people.
-Boil 1 tsp. of flaxseed in 1 c. water. Steep until lukewarm, then drink a cupful every 3-4 hours.
-Brew 3 T. peeled or cut up pumpkin seeds in 1 quart water for several hours. Drink 1/2 c. twice a day until relief is found.

AMISH FOLK MEDICINE

OTHER:
-Bladder infections (cystitis) are more likely in women and can be difficult to treat with continuous antibiotics. Cranberries, cranberry juice, and now a pill with extract of cranberry (see appendix) can be used to safely eliminate urinary tract infections.[45]

LEG ULCERS
-Apply a poultice of powdered sugar, lanolin, and tincture of benzoin. Massage the leg to improve circulation, rubbing upward.

LIVER
-Cook 5 medium size red beets in a quart of water. Drink the beet water and eat the beets (unpickled). Or boil the juice down to a smaller quantity and take a T. each morning before breakfast.

LOW BLOOD PRESSURE
-Fill a quart jar with finely diced beets, then add wine or whisky to the top of jar. Let stand 24 hours in warm place. Take 1-2 T. of this fluid twice daily.
-Eat plenty of fresh greens and red beets.
-Use blackstrap molasses often.

LUNG
-Take 1-2 capsules cayenne pepper with food in stomach to relieve pain of pleurisy.
-For pneumonia, make a chest salve by melting 1/2 lb. vaseline, 2 oz. gum camphor, 1/2 tsp. carbolic acid, and 1 T. beeswax. Another formula for chest salve: melt 6 oz. lard, 2 oz. pulverized camphor, and 3 oz. beeswax; followed by 3 oz. white resin, 2 oz. red balsam of Peru, 2 drams oil of cedar while stirring

AMISH FOLK MEDICINE

often. Apply this salve until begins to itch, then wash off with rubbing alcohol.
-Apply a poultice of equal parts flaxseed meal with ground black mustard to the chest.
-Drink hot pennyroyal tea.

MEASLES
-Eyes get weak during measles, so rest in a dark room and do not read.
-Boil a cup of oats in 4 cups of water for 15 minutes. Strain and sweeten. Drink at cool temperature.
-Drink tea made from yarrow.

MEMORY
-Eat hazel nuts for 9 days, beginning on first day by eating 6 nuts, then adding one extra nut each day.
-Eat green pepper seeds for 9 days beginning with 1 seed and doubling the dose until it reaches 256 seeds on the ninth day.
-Make a paste of ground cloves, peppers, dates, ginger, gulanga root, muskmelon seeds, and muscot nuts in equal quantities into olive oil. Eat 1 T. each morning before breakfast.
-Consume pills or make teas from the following herbs: chickweed, sweet flag, marigold, licorice root.
-Take 1 T. liquid lecithin daily.
-Get more lecithin by using Pam for frying foods.
-Eat muskmelon seeds.
    OTHER:
-Poor memory often results from decreased blood flow to the brain as we mature. Studies using 120 mg/day of ginkgo biloba extract dramatically improved blood flow and memory in older adults.[46]

AMISH FOLK MEDICINE

MENSTRUATION (abnormal, painful)
-Keep warm. Do not lift anything heavy. Don't eat anything with vinegar, lemon, lime, or grapefruit; or rich foods like candy bars and desserts.
-Drink tea made from blue cohosh.
-Drink tea made from 1/2 tsp. each of melissa tea with rue, steeped for 10 minutes, then strained.
-Chew fennel seeds to reduce pain.
-Drink a tea from pennyroyal daily beginning about 2 weeks before menstruation. Pennyroyal should not be consumed if pregnant.
-One of the oldest herbal concoctions consisted of: licorice, camomile, pleurisy root, Jamaica dogwood, black cohosh, life plant, and dandelion root in an alcohol tincture. Helps with both menopause and premenstrual syndrome. Used to be sold as Lydia Pinkham's tonic.
-Alternative formula: golden seal root, blessed thistle, cayenne, uva-ursi, cramp bark, false unicorn root, raspberry leaves, squaw vine, and ginger.
-To start monthly flow when there has been delayed menstruation, drink hot chamomile or ginger tea.
-For menstrual complaints of other nature, use tea from shave grass or horsetail grass.
-The whitish discharge from the vagina can be cleared up by administering a douche made of either 2 T. white vinegar or 2 tsp. alum per quart of lukewarm water.

MOOD
-Many Americans have a metabolism that is too high in acid from alcohol, soda pop, and coffee. Reduce acidity and return metabolism to more normal pH by

AMISH FOLK MEDICINE

eating more vegetables. Acidic people have a bitter and sour disposition.
-Take daily supplements of calcium (800 mg) and magnesium (800 mg).

MOTION SICKNESS
-Take 3-4 digestive enzymes 30 minutes before the trip.
    OTHER:
-Ginger tablets 30 minutes before the trip help many people with motion sickness.[47]
-By employing the time-tested effectiveness of acupressure points on the wrist, you can purchase (see appendix) elastic wrist bands with a small marble for the pressure point to relieve motion problems.

MOUTH SORES
-For sore mouth from dentures, make a cushioning poultice by soaking white lily flowers in whisky until petals look soaked. Use this mixture as a cushion between gums and dentures.
-Avoid all soda pop, which can be irritating. Make a mouth wash of 1 tsp. each powdered myrrh, golden seal, and cayenne pepper blended into 1 quart water. Rinse mouth daily.
-For canker sores, drink sage tea or apply pinch of powdered sage, goldenseal powder, or raw onion.
-For chapped lips, use lanolin lotion.
-L-lysine relieves mouth sores from viral herpes.
-Apply a poultice of extract of myrrh or sage.
-At first sign of mouth sores, gargle with a mixture of 1 tsp. soda and a pinch of salt in 1 c. warm water.

AMISH FOLK MEDICINE

-Wet the sore region, then dust with powdered golden seal or alum.

NERVE & SLEEP DISORDERS
-Eat light meals in the evening.
-Drink teas made from catnip, skullcap, peppermint, golden seal, black cohosh, or blue vervain before bedtime.
-Before retiring, rub the feet well with vinegar water.
-Replace fear with strength and confidence.
-Think no evil of your neighbor. Give love and love will be returned.
-Do not exalt yourself, as pride goes before the fall.
-Consider all the nice things that people do for you and what you can do for others.
-Think good thoughts that are pure, just, and honest.

NOSEBLEED
-To restrain the bleeding, press the nose firmly between the finger and thumb for a few minutes. Place a cold wet rag on the nape of the neck for a few minutes.
   OTHER:
-Nosebleeds can be caused by acute allergic reactions, such as from consuming milk, wheat, or other common allergenic foods.
-Use a cotton swab to apply Vicks to the inside of the nose to help prevent nosebleeds from dry winter weather.

OBESITY
-Temperance is the best prevention and cure. Eat less food and less often.

AMISH FOLK MEDICINE

-For 3 days, consume only fresh carrot juice. This will purge the body of toxins, rest the digestive tract, and encourage rapid weight loss. You may develop a slight orange tint to the skin, which is caused by the pigment beta-carotene. It is not harmful, and will fade within a few weeks.
-Drink Chinese slim tea daily.
-Notice how the more a person overeats, the further nature pushes that person away from the table.
-Eat only raw fruit and vegetables for 3 days to get started with quick results.
-To help avoid overeating, before each meal take 2 capsules of chickweed plus 2 capsules containing: saffron, burdock, parsley, kelp, licorice, fennel, echinacea, black walnut, papaya, hawthorn berries, and mandrake.
-Eat no sweets or baked products.
-To control appetite, drink a tea prepared from 1 tsp. of orange berries from the mountain ash tree.
-For 3 days, consume only pure unsweetened grape juice.
-Up to 25% of the population are underweight. For these people, take 10 drops daily of liquid red clover extract three times daily.
     OTHER:
-While calories do count, the most fat-inducing of calories is fat in the diet. Eat less fat and the weight will literally melt off your body.

PAIN
-Mix 1/4 oz. each of oil of organan, oil of hemlock, oil of lavender, oil of wintergreen, oil of cinnamon, oil of sassafras, with 1 oz. camphor gum, and 1 quart raw

AMISH FOLK MEDICINE

dietary linseed oil. Rub externally on burns, sores, sore throat, and other painful areas.

-For "tennis elbow", prepare a liniment by taking 4 fresh chopped avocado seeds, add 3 oz. horse tail grass to a quart of water and cook down to a pint. Add 1 pint of rubbing alcohol and bottle. Apply to sore area.

-For muscle soreness from long horse and buggy trips, soak in a hot tub for 3-5 minutes, then wrap in a warm blanket.

-Prepare a liniment known as "Good Samaritan Oil" by blending 1 quart raw linseed oil with 1/4 oz. oregano oil, 1/2 oz. oil of sassafras, 1/4 oz. wintergreen, 1/4 oz. oil of lavender, 1 oz. gum camphor. Gently rub on chest for colds.

-For back pain, mix 2 tablespoons cayenne pepper in 1 pint cider vinegar and boil for ten minutes. Allow to cool. Apply while still warm.

-A skilled massage can relieve many forms of pain.

-Dissolve 24 aspirin tablets in 1 quart rubbing alcohol and rub liberally on sore spot.

-Apply a salve from red tiger balm in rubbing alcohol to the sore area.

-Boil 2 T. cayenne pepper in 1 pint of cider vinegar for 10 minutes. Apply this hot solution to sore areas.

-Mix 50 aspirin with 8 grams (about 1/4 oz) of wintergreen oil and 1 pint rubbing alcohol. Rub on sore muscles or backache.

-For sciatica, the patient should lie on back, keeping knees straight. Another family member should grab the ankle and raise one leg at a time as far up over the head as possible. Repeat 3 times, then increase repetitions and angle of movement as pain decreases. Do <u>not</u> do if too painful.

AMISH FOLK MEDICINE

-For sciatica, grip both hands on a branch or overhead pipe to get the entire body off the ground. Hang the body loosely for a few seconds to stretch the spine. Draw the knees up as far as possible several times then rest.

PARASITES & WORMS (See a doctor first.)

-Eat hulled pumpkin seeds followed with a laxative. Or cook 8 chopped pumpkin seeds in a c. of boiling water and drink as a tea. For children, you may add 1-2 tsp. peppermint tea for flavor.
-Eat sauerkraut juice or garlic capsules to kill intestinal worms.
-Eat 3-4 dried peaches each night before retiring.
-Heat common unsalted lard to body temperature and place a squirt in the rectum with a medicine dropper.
-Eat hot spicey chili con carne daily to purge worms.
-Keep fingernails cut short to avoid contaminating food.
-Entacyl is a drug store remedy that can cure a whole family of pin worms in one day.

PLEURISY

(inflammation of the lungs)
-Take 4 capsules filled with red cayenne pepper every hour until the pain ceases. Drink plenty of water or tea afterward. Discontinue if this irritates stomach.

PNEUMONIA (See a doctor first.)

-Grind an onion, add barley flour and vinegar to make a paste. Heat and spread on cloth. Apply to chest.

AMISH FOLK MEDICINE

-Melt in frying pan: 6 oz. fresh lard, 3 oz. white resin, 3 oz. bees wax. Remove from stove and blend in: 2 oz. camphor oil, 2 drams balsam Peru. Put all ingredients into kettle and heat until melted. Strain into jars and cover. Spread ingredients on cloth, fold over, then warm and apply to chest. Cover with thick flannel cloth. Keep poultice compress hot.
-Mix 2 T. lard, 2 T. flour, 1 tsp. soda, 1 tsp. black pepper, 1 tsp. mustard. Never put a plaster with mustard against the skin. Spread mixture on cloth and lay on chest, poultice side up.

POISON IVY & OAK
-Apply a poultice of powdered alum in vaseline.
-Bath the affected parts in sassafras tea.
-Apply a poultice of crushed jewelweed stems and leaves.
-Wash affected parts with tansy tea.
-Add 2 tsp. lobelia to 1 c. boiling water. Let stand and apply to affected area.
-Soak the affected parts in a solution of epsom salts for 30 minutes daily.
-Bathe the affected area with a warm solution of salt water.
-Boil a 2x4 inch section of sprig oak bark in 1 quart water for 5 minutes, then simmer for 1 hour. Apply to the affected area for relief of itching.
-Wash skin region with tea from sassafras, jewelweed, or broom sage herbs.
-Rub the inside of a banana, lemon, or orange skin on the affected parts.
-Apply Caladryl from the drugstore.

POISONING

AMISH FOLK MEDICINE

-Easiest way to treat is to induce vomiting by giving Ipecac from drugstore. Do not induce vomiting if patient is in convulsions or unconscious.
-*Be sure to keep the number of your nearest poison control center handy by the phone. Call 911 for emergencies.

POULTICE & BONE KNITTER

-Make a tea from: white oak bark, comfrey root, marshmallow root, mullein, black walnut hulls, gravel root, wormwood, lobelia, and scullcap. Drink daily to speed the healing of a broken bone.
-For sores and boils, apply a poultice of: 1/2 c. beeswax cut fine, 1 c. lard (goose is best), 1 tsp. powdered resin melted together slowly over the stove, then cooled.
-"Green Mountain Salve" Mix 1 oz. resin, 1 oz. beeswax, and 4 oz. mutton tallow. Heat until melted. Stir in 1 dram pulverized vertergris, allow to cool, then form into a roll about 3/4 inch in diameter. Apply to wounds.
-For a poultice that heals bruises; mix 1/2 lb. fresh lard, 3 oz. white resin, 2 drams balsam of Peru, 1/4 lb. beeswax, 2 oz. pulverized camphor. Melt ingredients slowly over low heat, allow to cool in jars.
-Drink comfrey tea 3 times daily while taking bone meal capsules daily.
-To draw poison out of a wound, make a poultice from 1/4 c. each (lump the size of an egg) of hog's lard, beeswax, rosin, and hard brown laundry soap shaved fine. Heat ingredients slowly in an iron kettle, dissolve, pour into a jar and cool until hard.
-Mix a poultice to draw out poisons: chaparral, comfrey, red clover blossoms, pine tar, mullein, beeswax, plantain, olive oil, mutton, tallow,

AMISH FOLK MEDICINE

chickweed, poke root. Apply to ulcers, burns, and boils.
-To help disinfect a wound, make a poultice of equal parts sulphur and alum. Sprinkle on broken skin.
-Apply a poultice of fresh crushed peach leaves to bruises.
-To help disinfect a wound, soak the sore in 1 gallon of hot water with 3 T. hardwood ashes stirred in.
-This remedy was used to save a badly injured leg that would have been amputated: 1 lb. finely pulverized resin, 1 lb. mutton tallow shaved fine, 2 oz. pure olive oil, 2 oz granulated sugar. Mix all ingredients cold, do not heat. Apply three times daily to the affected parts.
-Apply a grated raw potato, fig, carrot, red beet, or onion to a skin area for relief and healing.
-Mix 1 T. epsom salt with 2 T. lard and apply to skin.
-Finely grate raw red beets and fill a cheesecloth bag, then apply to skin area.
-Mix raw egg yolk with 1 tsp. sugar and apply to lump.
-To help reduce polyps, especially in the nose region, take 2 ginseng capsules and 2-5 grams/day of vitamin C.
-Fry 1/2 lb mutton tallow then strain. Hardboil 3 dozen eggs then mash fine. Mix tallow and eggs on stove and add 1/2 c. olive oil, 1.5 lb. unsalted butter, 3 handfuls each of water balsam, sage, rue, and wild horseradish. Apply mixture to cuts, burns, and sores.
-Mix one pound clover blossoms with 1 pound vaseline and heat in the hot sun or oven for one hour. Strain through cheesecloth and store in jar. Apply to chapped hands and teats.

AMISH FOLK MEDICINE

PREGNANCY

-An herb to avoid if you want to get pregnant is pennyroyal. It discourages conception.

-For calming a stressful pregnant woman: a tea made from black cohosh, cayenne, hops flowers, mistletoe, lobelia, scullcap, wood betany, valerian root, and lady's slipper.

-If labor is overdue and the baby is ready to come but labor has not begun, consume one c. of blue cohosh tea followed by one c. of squaw vine tea.

-Amish women tend to look on pregnancy as normal, rather than a burden. A minor complaint includes kidney trouble (or edema, fluid retention), which they remedy with diuretic teas like sweet fennel, watermelon seeds, parsley, or bearberry.

-Most Amish women take an herbal mixture throughout pregnancy consisting of: equal parts of red raspberry and squaw vine capsule, 1-3 daily. Others will use the loose tea, since it is cheaper.

-For the last 6 weeks of pregnancy, use an herbal mixture of: squaw vine, blessed thistle, black cohosh, false unicorn, red raspberry leaves, lobelia. Normal dosage is 1-2 capsules 3 times daily. Amish women claim that this herbal remedy helps in faster and easier delivery by providing elasticity to the pelvic and vaginal areas.

-Another formula which helps both mother and infant: horsetail grass, oat straw, comfrey, lobelia.

-To stop post-partum (after birth) hemorrhaging, take the herbs ergot or shepherd's purse.

-To reverse thinning hair after delivery, take 20 drops daily of red clover tops tincture.

    MISCARRIAGE:

AMISH FOLK MEDICINE

-To help avoid miscarriage, drink tea from 1/2 handful of red raspberry leaves in one c. of boiling water.

-To help avoid miscarriage, drink tea from false unicorn, golden seal root, squaw vine, and orange peel.

MORNING SICKNESS & NAUSEA:

-Eat 2 T. brewer's yeast, extra iron, bone meal, and vitamin E daily.

-To stop nausea, drink a tea made from one (only!!) peach leaf.

-Drink red raspberry tea.

-Eat a few soda crackers about 15 minutes before getting out of bed. Eat small amounts of crackers throughout the day to settle the stomach.

-Eat one cup of yogurt in the evening before retiring.

-For the nausea or morning sickness of pregnancy, drink a tea made from red raspberry, spearmint leaf, alfalfa leaf, lemon verbena, lemon balm, nettle leaf, fennel seed, lemon grass leaf, and stevia leaf.

LACTATION:

-To encourage milk supply, mother should drink 1 quart of catnip tea daily. This calms both mother and infant.

-Marshmallow, or blessed thistle, or alfalfa tea help with mother's milk supply.

-For improved milk output, eat oatmeal gruel three times daily.

-For improved milk output, drink a tea from: fennel seeds, spearmint leaf, coriander seeds, lemon verbena, anise seed, chamomile flower, borage tops, blessed thistle leaf, althea root, lemon grass leaf, stevia leaf, and fenugreek seed.

BREAST LUMPS:

AMISH FOLK MEDICINE

-Make a poultice from equal parts of wintergreen oil, olive, and spirits of turpentine (not same as commercial type). Do not use while pregnant or nursing.
-Make a poultice from equal parts of castor oil and oil of wintergreen (genuine, not synthetic). Do not use while pregnant or nursing.
-Avoid eating chocolate.
-Active pregnant women usually have an easier delivery than women who are sedentary and get overweight.

PROSTATE
-Drink tea from burdock (gletta).
-Drink strong peppermint tea every hour.
-Take an enema of warm water, coffee, or salt water.
-Make a tea daily from the silk of 6 ears of corn boiled then steeped for 10 minutes. Drink a c. three times daily. Also acts as a diuretic.
-Also, chew fresh roasted pumpkin seeds. Also acts as worm-killer (vermifuge). As an option, may take tablets of pumpkin seed oil.
-Tea from Pau d'Arco helps.
-Take 50-100 mg zinc supplements daily.
    OTHER:
-Herbs of saw palmetto (serenoa repens) have been clinically proven to reduce swollen prostate gland in humans.[48]

RHEUMATIC FEVER
-Take pure mixed natural vitamin E before breakfast each day.

RHEUMATISM & ARTHRITIS

AMISH FOLK MEDICINE

-Make an herbal tonic by cutting up 6 oranges, 6 lemons, 6 grapefruit, cook them (peeling and all), in 2 quarts of water, strain, then add 1/4 c. epsom salt. Let it cook down to 1 quart, then stand overnight. Take 1 T. 3 times daily.

-Do not eat sugar, pork, or strawberries.

-Often caused by food poisoning from nightshade family. Avoid egg plant, green peppers, tomatoes, and potatoes, which contain substances that are harmful to certain sensitive individuals.

-Make an herbal preparation from: yucca, comfrey root, chaparral, alfalfa, burdock root, buckthorn bark, black cohosh root, parsley, slippery elm bark, yarrow, chelated trace minerals, cayenne, and lobelia.

-Take capsules of Devil's claw leaves.

-Drink pure aloe vera juice, 3 oz. three times daily.

-Reduce fat in the diet to clear up back pains. Eat less eggs, beef, pork, and cheese.

-Take extra calcium as supplements.

-Consume extra vitamin C (1-5 grams).

-Apply a poultice of equal parts olive oil and ammonia.

-Mix 2 oz. wintergreen oil with 1 pint rubbing alcohol and rub along the spine.

-Make a tea from 1/2 oz. each burdock, dock root, sassafras bark, dandelion, and dwarf elder. Boil in 2 quarts of water down to 1 quart. Three times daily take 2 T.

-Mix the juice of 3 lemons with 1 pint cold water, 1/4 c. epsom salts, and pinch cream of tartar. Take 2 tsp. first thing in morning.

-Eat one pokeberry on day one. Eat two pokeberries on day two, and so on till reaching 5 berries each day.

AMISH FOLK MEDICINE

-Mix 3 oz. olive oil, 2 oz. charcoal, 1 lb. figs, 1.5 lb. raisins, 1 oz. glycerine, 3 oz. powdered senna, and 1 oz. slippery elm powder. Grind the fruit, then mix dry ingredients. Next add oil and glycerine. Mix with hands and form into walnut size balls. Take one lump in morning and one in evening for first week. Afterward, take only one lump in evening and none in morning.

-Add 4-10 bone meal tablets daily to the diet, especially for back pain.

-Pour 1 quart boiling water over 6 T. alfalfa seeds and steep for 15 minutes. Drink 2 cups daily, morning and evening, beginning with only 1/2 c. twice daily.

-Take 1 tsp. cod liver oil daily, washed down with unsweetened fruit juice.

-Drink goat's milk.

-Prepare 6 lemons squeezed and cut up, 1 pint alfalfa honey, 1 small can cream of tartar, 1 tsp. epsom salts in 1 quart boiling water. Let stand overnight. Strain and keep refrigerated. Take 1 T. in morning and another T. at night.

-Eat one boiled lemon each day for 50 days.

-Mix 1 tsp. cider vinegar in 1 glass tomato juice and drink 2 or more glasses daily, preferably before meals on an empty stomach.

-Dissolve 1/2 tsp. epsom salts in 2 cups water which has been boiled then cooled. Add the juice of 2 lemons, then pour into a glass jar and keep refrigerated. Take 2 T. each morning before breakfast. Aspirin along with this remedy may help ease pain.

-Take 50-100 mg. zinc daily.

AMISH FOLK MEDICINE

-If symptoms are actually from gout, abstain from red meat.
-Mix 1 pint gin, 2 oz. juniper berries, 1 T. epsom salts, and 1 T. sugar. Take 1 tsp. 3 times daily.
-Pack quart can with ferns then fill with rubbing alcohol and set in sun for 4 weeks. Rub this lotion on ailing parts.

RINGWORM
-Apply a poultice of 2 parts lard and 1 part sulphur to the affected area. Use old clothes, for this poultice will soil clothes.
-Hold an icepack to the sore for 5-10 minutes.
-Wash the area or hair with tar soap and borax, then moisten the spots with a solution from 1/2 tsp. golden seal, 1/2 tsp. myrrh, and 1 tsp. bloodroot that has been steeped in a pint of boiling water.
-Drink at least one c. daily of tea from golden seal.

SEX DESIRE
-Chew on ginseng root daily.
-An herbal combination used often by the Amish for men over 40 includes: Damiana, Siberian ginseng, echinacea, Fo-Ti, Gotu-Kola, sarsaparilla, and saw palmetto.
    OTHER:
-Married men live 5 years longer than bachelors. Men who kiss their wives daily live an average of 5 years longer than married men who do not regularly kiss their wives. British widowers have a 40% higher heart attack death rate than their married peers.
-Thyroid. 40% or more of the population suffers from low thyroid output (hypothyroidism), especially as we age. Low thyroid can influence many processes,

including sex drive[49]. Recommendation: if your basal temperature first thing in the morning is below 97.8 F, then you are a likely candidate for thyroid supplementation. Work with your doctor, since thyroid is a prescription medication. As an option, you can stimulate the thyroid gland by providing the proper raw ingredients for its functioning, including iodine (10 drops liquid kelp) and 15 drops of thyroid stimulant from Natural Herbal Extract (see appendix).

SHINGLES
-May be caused by nervousness, so consume more B vitamins and nerve tonic teas.
-Take up to 6 grams daily of L-lysine.
-Apply a hot cloth soaked in a solution of pine bark and mulberry leaves.

SINUS CONGESTION
(see also "colds")
-See "allergy" section for nasal purge with salt water.
-To relieve sinus congestion of colds and flu, add peppermint or spearmint oil to a vaporizer at night.
-Place a pinch of goldenseal on the tongue.
-Drink goldenseal tea while eliminating all dairy products from the diet.
-Mix handful of pennyroyal leaves in 6 oz. sweet almond oil until the oil turns green, then add a few grams of horehound powder. Use a few drops of this mixture in the nose for decongestion.
-To cut down on bacteria count in the air, add pine, cedar, or mint oil in a vaporizer. Europeans have long known that a sanitorium in an evergreen forest is more conducive to recuperation. Some hospitals

AMISH FOLK MEDICINE

would bring potted pine trees into the rooms to help patients recover.
-Use the Olbas inhaler from Switzerland, containing oils of menthol, peppermint, and eucalyptol.
-Rub outside of nose area with Vicks before retiring.
-Mix 1 quart water, 1/4 c. vinegar, and 2 T. honey. Drink 1 c. of this solution daily.
-Use an eye dropper to apply a small amount of warm mineral oil (baby oil) in the nose with head hung over bed to keep solution in nose.
-Mix 2 cups water and 2 T. vinegar in a kettle and boil. Put a towel over your head and around the kettle in order to inhale the steam. Do this for 5-10 minutes daily.
-Mix 1 c. warm water, 1/4 tsp. salt, 1/4 tsp. listerine. Use as nasal purge described in "allergy" section.
-Drink tea or chew sections from angelica root.
-Mix 1 pint water, 1 tsp. salt, 1 tsp. peppermint oil, 1 tsp. boric acid, 1 tsp. baking soda and use as nasal purge described in "allergy" section.
-Drink tea from mullein.
   OTHER:
-While many Americans take antibiotics for a cold, antibiotics do nothing for a viral infection and may reduce the immune system's ability to fight the cold. Only take medication when it is absolutely necessary.

SPRAINS
-Immediately after the injury, apply cold towels to the site (to reduce swelling). Next day alternate between cold and hot applications. Third day use hot towels (to improve healing).
-Apply a hot poultice of vinegar.

AMISH FOLK MEDICINE

-Fry black root in lard, cool and rub it on the sprained part.
-Drink boneset tea.

SPURS
-Take supplements of calcium and magnesium (800 mg. each).
-Wear good arch supports in your shoes.

STOMACH PROBLEMS
-Eat an occasional soda cracker.
-Every morning before breakfast, drink a glass of hot water with 2 tsp. cider vinegar and 2 tsp. honey.
-Chew caraway seeds for an upset stomach.
-Each morning drink a tea made from 1/4 tsp. sage or golden seal in 1 c. hot water.
-Mix "go back" drops by combining 1 oz. glycerine, 10 drops aconite tincture, and 1 oz. rain water. Take 3-5 drops twice daily for 3 days. Wait 3 days and repeat dose.
-For heartburn, drink 1/4 c. water with 1/4 tsp. baking soda.
-Drink tea from burdock root.
-For pain in stomach, be aware of foods that may cause an allergy.
-Drink a tea made from golden seal one hour before mealtime. Other helpful teas for stomach problems include: thyme, cayenne, fennel, ginseng, sage, sassafras, slippery elm, and chickweed.
-For stomach ulcer, consume 2 T. sauerkraut juice before eating.
-Mix 1 T. mutton tallow in a half c. of hot milk taken 30 minutes before mealtime and followed by a glass of cold water.

AMISH FOLK MEDICINE

-To build stomach muscles and get rid of bulging stomach, lie flat on back on padded floor. Raise both feet slowly, keeping knees straight, as high as is comfortable, then lower almost to the floor; and repeat this exercise. Start slowly with 4-5 repetitions, then build up to higher repetitions.

STROKE
-To help encourage recovery in the damaged tissue, use physical therapy and bath the affected body parts with tea made from cayenne pepper and water.

SWEATY FEET
-Wear white cotton stockings.
-Bathe feet frequently.
-For feet that do not sweat, walk through morning dew in bare feet, then rub feet vigorously with towel.
-To squelch foot odor, sprinkle baking soda powder inside shoes.
-For tired feet, soak feet for 20 minutes in solution of 1 quart hot water with 1 tsp. boric acid.

THROAT
-For dry throat common in speakers, chew small pieces of dried calamus root.
-Chew a piece of ginseng root.
-Take 1 tsp. Olba's Oil, found in health food stores.
-For strep throat, apply a poultice of grated garden beets on the outside of the throat. Freshen poultice when the beets will turn a greenish color. Continue changing and applying this poultice until the beets do not change color.
-Suck on fresh cloves of garlic.
-Take 10 drops 2-3 times daily of red clover tops.

AMISH FOLK MEDICINE

-For swollen throat glands, gargle with a mixture of 7 lime rinds boiled in milk.
-For swollen glands, apply a piece of flannel soaked in warm vinegar. Do not squeeze glands!!
-Drink tea from mullein and lobelia.
-For hoarseness, beat stiff the white of a fresh egg. Add juice of one lemon, 1 T. glycerine, 1 tsp. sugar. Take a swallow often until hoarseness disappers.
-For tonsillitis, gargle with tea from red clover tops. Externally apply a poultice of onions. Or take thymus extract, available from health food store. Or make an herbal preparation from equal parts scullcap, lobelia, valerian root, myrrh, gum, black cohosh, and cayenne.

TOBACCO HABIT (to quit)
-For several days, drink only unsweetened fruit and vegetable juices to cleanse the system.
-Take a relaxing hot bath each day.
-Drink tea from red clover for cleansing.
-Drink tea from gentian, magnolia, or catnip to reduce cravings.

TONIC (purifier, energizer, toner)
-Boil down 1/2 ounce of Snake Root (Aristolochia serpentaria) in a pint of boiling water for 2 hours. Take 1 tsp. three times daily.
-Eat watercress, alfalfa sprouts, or dandelion leaves in a salad.
-Make homemade gingerale by chopping up a fresh ginger root in a quart of water. Simmer until water is yellow, strain, add honey and carbonated water.
-Soak 3 quarts of dandelion flowers in 2 quarts of water for 3 days. Strain, add 2 pounds sugar, 1

AMISH FOLK MEDICINE

sliced lemon, 1 T. yeast; then let stand for 4 days and bottle it. Use 1 T. before each meal.
-Take 2 oz. each of sarsaparilla root, sassafras root, spikenard root, black birch bark, yellow dock root, and spruce needles. Boil in 4 gallons of water for 25 minutes, strain, let cool. Add 1 lb. brown sugar and 3 T. yeast and let it ferment (allow escape valve for gases). Bottle after 3 days. Drink a c. as needed.
-Pick fresh stinging nettles with a leather glove. Boil 1 oz. in 1 pint of water and take 1 T. daily.

TONSILLITIS
-Mix 1 T. yellow root, 1/2 tsp. salt, 1 tsp. garden sage, 1/2 tsp soda. Simmer in 1 c. water for 30 minutes, then cool and add 1/2 c. cider vinegar. Gargle every few hours with this solution.
-Swab the tonsils with a cotton swab dipped in 1/2 oz. iodine mixed with 1/2 oz. glycerine.
-Mix 1 T. yellow dock root, 1 tsp. garden sage, 1/2 tsp salt, 1/2 tsp soda in 1 c. water then cool and add 1/2 c. cider vinegar. Gargle with this solution every 3 hours.
-At first sign of oncoming sore throat, take a tsp. of honey every hour.
-Sip the juice of 1 lemon mixed with 1 tsp. honey. May be added to hot water for tea mixture.
-Put a peeled and cleaned garlic bulb in the mouth and bite on it regularly. Discomfort will lessen.
-Make a gargle solution with 4 oz water, 1/2 tsp. salt and 1/2 tasp soda.
-Make a gargle solution with 1 c. hot water, 1 tsp. vinegar, and sprinkling of hot pepper powder. Gargle every 15 minutes.

AMISH FOLK MEDICINE

TOOTHACHE & TEETH
-Cut down on dental bills by adding bone meal and wheat germ to baked bread and cookies. Builds strong teeth.
-Eat asparagus everyday (fresh or canned) and you will either have no problems, or be able to bear the pain until you can get to a dentist.
-Soak cotton in oil of clove and place next to sore tooth.
-Cut fresh fig in half and lay next to sore tooth.
-Drink tea from equal parts: horsetail grass, comfrey root, oat straw, and lobelia.
-Fry an onion until hot then pour into a small cloth bag. If the toothache is on the right side of the mouth, then place the bag on the pulse of the right wrist region. If the toothache is on the left side of the mouth, then place the bag on the pulse of the left wrist region.
-Place ice on the sore tooth.
-Fill the tooth cavity with a small cotton plug soaked in cayenne, peppermint oil, and aspirin.
-Sugar is expensive: you pay for it twice; once at the grocery store and again at the dentist.

ULCER & COLITIS
-Drink 6 oz of cabbage juice a half hour before meals. Prepare juice by placing 3 cups of chopped cabbage in a blender with 16 oz water, then strain.
-Take capsules of comfrey and fenugreek.
-Take capsules of the following combination: slippery elm, comfrey root, lobelia, ginger, and wild yam.
-Eat a bit of cabbage with each meal, chewing slowly.
-Drink golden seal tea.

AMISH FOLK MEDICINE

-Consume only grapes or grape juice for 3 days. Must be in good health to attempt this fast.
-Drink glass of aloe vera daily.

VARICOSE VEINS
-Drink 3 cups daily of white oak bark tea.
-To strengthen the muscles and blood vessels in the leg region, jump rope daily, but begin slowly (1 minute) and build up to 5 minutes.
-Eat plenty of fresh garlic and take vitamin E supplements.
-To relieve the pain, bathe the legs in vinegar 3 times daily.
-For ulcers that form on varicose veins, apply dry powdered sugar.

VINEGAR
-Vinegar has so many uses and is so cheap and non-toxic that it merits its own section.
-Use vinegar for an underarm deodorant after bathing.
-Use vinegar diluted in a glass of warm water as a gargle for sore throat.
-Soak soiled clothes in vinegar to remove stubborn stains.
-Rub vinegar on insect stings.
-Use vinegar as hair rinse.
-Rinse diapers in vinegar to help prevent diaper rash.
-In hot water, rinse with vinegar for a cooling sensation.
-Boil vinegar in pot on stove and inhale vapors to clear plugged sinuses.

AMISH FOLK MEDICINE

-To help prevent food poisoning when visiting foreign countries or questionable restaurants, take 1 T. vinegar in a glass of water 30 minutes before eating.

WARTS
-Soak a bandage in castor oil and tie around wart region.
-Apply celandine or milkweed juice.
-Touch the wart with a toothpick soaked in castor oil. Also helps to eliminate corns.
-Rub wart with raw potato peelings.
-Wash wart region 3 times daily with baking soda and water solution.
-Apply the milky juice of a dandelion to the wart.
-Rub the wart each day with a piece of white chalk.
-Apply the juice from milkweed to the wart.
-Apply wood ashes to the wart.
-Apply iodine daily.
-Rub garlic on wart daily.

AMISH FOLK MEDICINE

APPENDIX A
SOURCES: WHERE TO BUY

Herbs & Vitamins:
-Chupp's Herbs & Vitamins, 27539 Londick, Burr Oak, MI 49030-9746
-East-West Herbs, 65 Mechanic St. #103, Red Bank, NJ; ph 800-542-6544
-Planetary Formulas, Box 533W, Soquel, CA 95073; ph 800-776-7701
-Nature's Herbs, Box 118, Norway, IA 52318; ph.800-365-4372
-Enzymatic Therapy, 510 Lombardi Ave., Greenbay, WI 54304; ph.800-558-7372
-Bronson Pharmaceuticals, 4526 Rinetti Lane, La Canada, CA 91011-0628; ph. 800-235-3200
-Min Tong Herbs, 3252 Ramona St., Pinole, CA 94564; ph. 800-538-1333

Easy to take powder vitamin C:
-Seraphim, 800-553-5472

Cranberry extract pills:
-Ecological Formulas, Concord, CA, ph. 800-888-4585

Special Natural Vitamin E:
-A.C. Grace Company,1100 Quitman Rd, Big Sandy, TX 75755; ph. 903-636-4368

Special mixture of EPA (fish oil) and GLA (borage oil):

AMISH FOLK MEDICINE

-BioSyn, Inc., 21 Tioga Way, Marblehead, MA 01945; ph. 800-346-2703

Aloe vera with active ingredient:
Royal Body Care, 10575 Newkirk
Dallas, TX 75220; ph. 214-401-0052

Salve for sun spots on skin:
-Cansema, Applied Botanical Research, Box 350, Lake Charles, LA 70602-0350; ph. 800-256-2253

Wrist Band to relieve motion sickness:
-Solutions, Box 6878, Portland, OR 97228; ph.800-342-9988

Amish Life and Christian Education:
-Basic Christian Education, Box D, Nottawa, MI 49075

AMISH FOLK MEDICINE

APPENDIX B
WHAT IS A HEALTHY LIFESTYLE?

Many of the recommendations listed in this book assume that the person is already living a healthy lifestyle, like the Amish, and has eliminated many possible causative factors for their symptoms. Not only is the "healthy lifestyle" not taught in American schools, but we are continuously bombarded with commercials for expensive "junk food and drink". Even our physicians are woefully unprepared on the subject of nutrition and healthy lifestyle.

This section is included for a good reason: you can take the home remedies recommended in the earlier part of this book, but if you are obese, sedentary, stressed, smoking, drinking, and doing other major factors wrong, then a little herb tea will be unable to reverse all the negative forces from your lifestyle. Hence, it is crucial that you follow this section PLUS do whatever the book recommends for your symptoms.

I have found it unwise to lay out a detailed food and exercise program for people. By the second day, he or she will be out of a food item, or eat a their aunt's house and just discard the program altogether. However, when you become your own nutritionist, then you can take that good judgment into any unforeseen circumstances and make a good decision. Navigational school for sailors does not include an escort around the world to show people how to find everything. Instead, you are taught how to use a sextant, compass, and map; and from those

AMISH FOLK MEDICINE

tools you can find your way anywhere, because you now have good judgment. Similarly, I can't follow you around for the rest of your life and tell you what is best for your health, but I can implant good judgment with a few simple rules. Consider these rules your "sextant, compass, and map" to steer clear of the rocky shoals of unhealthy lifestyle and toward the clear open seas of healthy practices. Good luck and good sailing!!

A HEALTHY LIFESTYLE INCLUDES:

1) Optimal nutrition. See the "Cardinal Rules" listed below.
2) Regular exercise. To include stretching, strengthening, and aerobic conditioning. At the very least, take a brisk 30 minute walk daily. For even better results, join a fitness club, or get a stair climber or cross country skiing device, or simply follow any of the dozens of workout videos available at your local video store. Of course, see your doctor before beginning any exercise program.
3) Toxin avoidance. Your body is constantly working to excrete the toxic by-products of living through feces, urine, and sweat. In our heavily polluted industrial age, too many people are exposed to overwhelming amounts of additional air, water, and food pollutants that tax the body's ability to eliminate poisons. Get a water filter device for your kitchen sink. If you live in a polluted region, get politically involved and clean up the air or move. Soak your fresh produce in a mild solution of warm water and 1/4 c. of vinegar for 5 minutes, rinse, then eat as usual. For more on improving your body's ability to tolerate toxins, see my book SAFE EATING.

AMISH FOLK MEDICINE

4) Attitude. For centuries, mystics, religious leaders, and philosophers have told us about the link between the mind and body. An abundance of research shows that the most blatant risk factor toward heart disease is loneliness. There are textbooks with thousands of scientific references showing the important link between mind and the major killers and cripplers in Western society: heart disease, cancer, diabetes, allergies, osteoporosis, mental illness, infections, etc. Scientists have found that our immune factors; which are "tiny soldiers" that patrol the body to destroy invading bacteria, virus, or cancer cells; have receptors for brain chemicals (neurochemical transmitters). Think about that!! Each of our vital protective soldiers has a "nervous system" of sorts. When you are depressed, so is your immune system. Think love, joy, beauty, and forgiveness. Find something that you would do for free and figure out a way to be paid for it. Have someone to love, something to do, and something to look forward to.

Or "...whatever is honorable, whatever is right, whatever is pure, whatever is lovely, whatever is of good repute, if there is any excellence and if anything worthy of priase, let your mind dwell on these things." (Philippians 4:19).

5) Body maintenance. Wear comfortable shoes with good arch support, wide toes, and breathable leather. Use a mattress that provides support without being too hard. Adjustable inflatable air mattresses are wonderful. Use a small pillow in the small part (lumbar) of your back when you sit for extended periods. Whenever possible, lie on the floor with the lower part of your legs up on a footstool to improve

AMISH FOLK MEDICINE

leg circulation. Wear a hat and use sunglasses and sunscreen lotion when in the sun. Use foam ear protectors when around loud noises. Many of these recommendations may seem obvious to some of you, but too many people expect this mortal body to withstand endless abuse and neglect. With care, your body is built to last 8 or 10 decades with dependable service.

CARDINAL RULES OF NUTRITION

-Eat foods in as close to their natural state as possible. Biochemists discover something new everyday to support this statement. Think of the "Divine design" that went into creating our food supply. For minimally processed foods, shop the perimeter of the grocery store.

-Eat a wide variety of foods. While there are some very nutrient-dense foods that should be included often in your diet, there are no perfect foods that have all the essential nutrients. By eating various plant and animal foods, you are much more likely to include essential but poorly understood nutrients.

-Eat small frequent meals, relying more on 4-6 small snacks per day rather than 1-3 huge meals.

-Minimize intake of fat, salt, sugar, cholesterol, alcohol, and caffeine. Avoid processed meats (luncheon, smoked, salted) and food additives (especially nitrites, MSG, and food colorings).

-Maximize intake of fresh vegetables, fruit, whole grains, beans, fish, poultry, low fat dairy, and clean water. These should constitute the "staples" of your diet. Mentally cut up your dinner plate into pie sections where 2/3 is unprocessed plant food and

AMISH FOLK MEDICINE

1/3 is lowfat high protein animal food. This is the ancestral diet for most humans.

-For people who eat meat, select animals that used to fly, swim, or run. Cows are locked in stationary positions to build fat and weight quicker. Minimize beef intake.

> **-FINALLY, AS AN OVERALL TEST OF YOUR FOOD: IF IT WILL NOT SPROUT OR ROT, THEN DON'T EAT IT. BECAUSE IF THE FOOD CANNOT NOURISH A BACTERIA CELL, THEN IT CANNOT NOURISH YOUR BODY CELLS EITHER.**

-Get your nutrients "with a fork and spoon" through food. Realistically, due to stress, pollution, sedentary lives, and junk food, we cannot obtain optimal amounts of nutrients through food alone. Hence, a quality broad spectrum vitamin mineral supplement is valuable for all people and essential for most people. The following is a list of nutrients that should be taken regularly to help reduce the incidence and severity of disease, delay the aging process, and improve vitality, fertility, and awareness. You can find a broad spectrum vitamin similar to this list available from several vendors listed in the appendix or at your health food store.

AMISH FOLK MEDICINE

NUTRIENT	SUPPLEMENTAL RANGE
Vitamins:	
A (beta-carotene)	10,000-25,000 iu
D (cholecalciferol)	400-800 iu
E (mixed natural tocopherols)	800-2400 iu
K (phytonadione)	100-1000 mcg
B-1 (thiamin)	4-50 mg
B-2 (riboflavin)	4-50 mg
B-3 (niacinamide)	20-200 mg
B-6 (pyridoxine)	6-50 mg
B-12 (cobalamin)	12-1000 mcg
folacin (folic acid)	400-800 mcg
biotin (biotin)	300-600 mcg
C (ascorbic acid)	500-5000 mg
pantothenic acid	30-100 mg
choline (as bitartrate)	250-500 mg
Minerals:	
calcium (ionized, or citrate)	400-800 mg
magnesium (ionized, or citrate)	400-800 mg
zinc (picolinate)	15-50 mg
iron (chelated)	10-30 mg
copper (chelated)	1-3 mg
iodine (potassium iodide)	150-1000 mcg
manganese (chelated)	5-10 mg
chromium (picolinate, or yeast)	200-400 mcg
molybdenum (chelated)	150-300 mcg
selenium (selenomethionine)	200-400 mcg
silicon (Mg-trisilicate)	10-20 mg
vanadium (Na-metavanadate)	10-20 mcg
EPA (fish oil)	1-2 T., or 3-6 caps

APPENDIX C
REFERENCES

PRIMARY TEXTBOOKS; EXCELLENT GENERAL READING

Carper, J., THE FOOD PHARMACY, Bantam Books, NY, 1988
Gottlieb, W. (ed.), DOCTORS BOOK OF HOME REMEDIES, Rodale Press, Emmaus, PA, 1990
Hausman, P., & Hurley, JB, HEALING FOODS, Dell, NY, 1989
Jarvis, DC, FOLK MEDICINE, Fawcett Crest, NY, 1958
Kaptchuk, T., & Croucher, M., THE HEALING ARTS, Summit Books, NY, 1987
Kerr, RW, HERBALISM THROUGH THE AGES, Kingsport Press, Kingsport, TN, 1969
Langer, SE, SOLVED THE RIDDLE OF ILLNESS, Keats, New Canaan, CT, 1984
Lau, BL, GARLIC FOR HEALTH, Lotus Light, Wilmot WI, 1988
Lieberman, S., & Bruning, N., THE REAL VITAMIN & MINERAL BOOK, Avery, NY, 1990
Lucas, R., SECRETS OF THE CHINESE HERBALISTS, Parker Publ, W. Nyack NY, 1977
Lust, J., THE HERB BOOK, Bantam Books, NY, 1974
McGrath, W., AMISH FOLK REMEDIES, Freeport Press, 1985
Meyer, C., AMERICAN FOLK MEDICINE, Meyerbooks, Glenwood, IL, 1985
Mowrey, DB, SCIENTIFIC VALIDATION OF HERBAL MEDICINE, Keats, New Canaan, CT, 1986
Murray, MT, HEALING POWER OF HERBS, Prima, Sacramento, 1991
Murray, MT, & Pizzorno, J., ENCYCLOPEDIA OF NATURAL MEDICINE, Prima, Sacramento, 1990
Quillin, P, HEALING NUTRIENTS, Random House, NY, 1987
Rinzler, CA, FEED A COLD, STARVE A FEVER, Facts on File, NY, 1991

Royal, PC, HERBALLY YOURS, Sound Nutrition, Hurricane UT, 1982
Tierra, M, THE WAY OF HERBS, Pocket Books, NY, 1990
Weaver, SM, GRANDMA'S HOME REMEDIES, Fani's Books, Millersburg, OH 1988
Weiner, M., WEINER'S HERBAL, Quantum Books, Mill Valley, CA, 1990
Werbach, M., NUTRITIONAL INFLUENCES ON ILLNESS, Third Line Press, Tarzana, CA, 1993

OTHER SELECTED SCIENTIFIC REFERENCES:

[1]. Quillin, P., HEALING NUTRIENTS, Random House, NY, 1987

[2]. Random House Encyclopedia, Random House, p.745, NY, 1983

[3]. Murray, MT, HEALING POWER OF HERBS, p.1, Prima Publ, Sacramento, 1991

[4]. THE COMPLETE DRUG REFERENCE, p.372, Consumers Union, Yonkers, NY, 1992

[5]. Duke, JA, HANDBOOK OF MEDICINAL HERBS, p.78, CRC Press, Boca Raton, FL, 1985; see also Leung, AY, ENCYCLOPEDIA OF COMMON NATURAL INGREDIENTS USED IN FOOD, DRUGS, AND COSMETICS, p.52, John Wiley Press, NY, 1980

[6]. Nassar, BA, et al., Nutrition Research, vol.6, p.1397, 1986

[7]. Downing, DT, et al., Journal of the American Academy of Dermatology, vol.14, p.221, 1986

[8]. Schachner, L, Pediatric Clinics of North America, vol.30, p.337, 1980

[9]. Cunliffe, J, British Journal of Dermatology, vol.101, p.321, 1979

[10]. Verna, KC, et al., Acta Dermatovener, vol.60, p.337, 1980

[11]. Elias, PM, et al., Archives of Dermatology, vol.117, p.160, Mar.1981; see also International Journal of Dermatology, vol.20, p.278, 1981

[12]. McCarty, M, Medical Hypotheses, vol.14, p.307, 1984

[13]. Michaelsson, G., et al., Acta Dermto-Venerologica, vol.64, p.9, 1984

[14]. Hendler, SS, THE DOCTORS' VITAMIN AND MINERAL ENCYCLOPEDIA, Simon & Schuster, NY, 1990; see also Davies, S., & Stewart, A., NUTRITIONAL MEDICINE, Avon, NY, 1987

[15]. Werbach, MR, NUTRITIONAL INFLUENCES ON ILLNESS, p.23-38, Third Line Press, Tarzana, 1992

[16]. Williams, RJ, THE PREVENTION OF ALCOHOLISM THROUGH NUTRITION, Bantam, NY, 1981

[17]. Krohn, J., ALLERGY RELIEF AND PREVENTION, Hartley & Marks, Pt. Roberts, WA, 1991

[18]. Burr, ML, et al., Human Nutrition: Applied Nutrition, vol. 39A, p.349, Oct.1985; see also Pelikan, Z. et al., Annals of Allergy, vol.58, p.164, Mar.1987

[19]. Koepke, JW, et al., Annals of Allergy, vol.54, p.213, Mar.1985

[20]. Reynolds, RD, et al., Federation Proceedings, vol.43, p.470, 1984

[21]. Mohsenin, L., et al., American Review of Respiratory Disease, vol.127, p.143, 1983

[22]. Okayama, H., et al., Journal of American Medical Association, vol.257, p.1076, Feb.27, 1987

[23]. Balch, JF, & Balch, PA, PRESCRIPTION FOR NUTRITIONAL HEALING, p.100, Avery, NY, 1990

[24]. Murray, M., & Pizzorno, J., ENCYCLOPEDIA OF NATURAL MEDICINE, p.56, Prima, Sacramento, 1990

[25]. Crook, WG, HELP FOR THE HYPERACTIVE CHILD, Professional Books, Jackson, TN, 1991

[26]. Machlin, LJ, HANDBOOK OF VITAMINS, p.145, Marcel Dekker, NY, 1991

[27]. Hendler, SS, ibid, p.247

[28]. Werbach, M., ibid, p.47

[29]. Quillin, P., in Hetter (ed.), LIPOPLASTY, p.209, Little, Brown, Boston, 1990

[30]. Whitaker, J., Health & Healing, Vol.3, no.1, p.4, Jan.1993

[31]. Werbach, M., ibid, p.196

[32]. Hendler, SS, ibid, p.87
[33]. Eby, GA, et al., Antimicrobial Agents & Chemotherapy, vol.25, p.20, 1984
[34]. Lewin, S., VITAMIN C: ITS MOLECULAR BIOLOGY AND MEDICAL POTENTIAL, NY, Van Nostrand Reinhold, 1973
[35]. Terezhalmy, GT, et al., Oral Surgery, vol.45, p.56, 1978
[36]. Starasoler, S. et al., NY State Dental Journal, vol.44, no.9, p.382, 1978
[37]. Griffith, RS, Dermatologica, vol.175, p.183, 1987
[38]. Quillin, P., ibid, p.344
[39]. Quillin, P., ibid, p.294
[40]. Budoff, PW, NO MORE HOT FLASHES, Warner, NY 1983
[41]. Werbach, MR, ibid, p.376
[42]. Johnson, ES, et al., British Medical Journal, vol.291, p.569, Aug.1985
[43]. Quillin, P., ibid, p.81
[44]. Leathwood, P., et al., Pharmacological Biochemistry Behavior, vol.17, p.65, 1982; see also Leathwood, P, et al., Planta Medica, vol.54, p.144, 1985
[45]. Prodromos, PN, et al., Southwest Medicine, vol.47, p.17, 1968; see also Sternlieb, P., New England Journal Medicine, vol.268, p.57, 1963
[46]. Vorberg, G., Clinical Trials Journal, vol.22, p.149, 1985
[47]. Mowrey, D. et al., Lancet, vol.i, p.655, 1982
[48]. Champlault, G, et al., British Journal Clinical Pharmacology, vol.18, p.461, 1984
[49]. Langer, SE, SOLVED: THE RIDDLE OF ILLNESS, p.40, Keats, New Canaan, CT, 1984